Hope Within Me

For Shelly,

may you always
know the power of grace &
love within friends, family,
and most importantly God.
Even our darkest moments,
for that's where we meet
with Him.

"And surely I am with you
always, to the very end of
the age."
          - Matthew 28:20

Hope Within Me

A Memoir of

Friendship, Courage,

Overcoming Struggle,

& Healing

. . . . . .

JAMES VALENCIA

[signature]

4-27-21   author HOUSE

AuthorHouse™
1663 Liberty Drive
Bloomington, IN 47403
www.authorhouse.com
Phone: 833-262-8899

Published by AuthorHouse 01/08/2021

ISBN: 978-1-6655-1287-9 (sc)
ISBN: 978-1-6655-1288-6 (hc)
ISBN: 978-1-6655-1314-2 (e)

Library of Congress Control Number: 2021900339

For my family and friends

AUTHOR'S NOTE

During the ten years since my diagnosis with Epilepsy, I never would have imagined the road it would have taken me down. So many tears, trials, and frustrations. The many AEDs (anti-Epileptic drugs) I tried, working only to fail later. All the different neurologists, Epileptologists, physicians, and appointments at various locations, as well as the hospitalizations I needed. The many diagnosis I received sending me into sadness, depression, anger, and hopelessness at times. At the same time, the many unforgettable friends, colleagues, and doctors I met along the way I wouldn't trade for anything. Just like any memoir, the chronology, and conversations of this is accurate, altered only when necessary. I have excluded certain details that seemed irrelevant to the nature of the story. The identity of places and key figures in my life are changed, for instance: Miss Evans, Doctor Michaels, Breezy, Doctor Klark, Dr. Marino, Dr. Anders, Dr. Bailey, Tina, Kris, Ted, Steven, Mira, Jeff, Doctor Devrat, Doctor Boden.

In all, I wish I were never diagnosed or any of this had happened to me. Maybe my life would have been better. But at times, as difficult as it was, I thank God for what took place.

"Dear Epilepsy, just so you know, I won't give up. I won't give in. I have endless hope. Endless faith. You may be in my life. But you don't own my life."

"We don't know how strong we are until being strong is the only choice we have."

"Epilepsy changes people. It sculpts us into someone who understands more deeply, hurts more often, appreciates more quickly, cries more easily, hopes more desperately, loves more openly, and lives more passionately."

BACKGROUND INFORMATION

ABOUT

EPILEPSY & SEIZURES

Epilepsy by The Numbers

- **65 million** people around the world live with Epilepsy.

- **3.4 million** people in the U.S. live with Epilepsy.

  Approx. **470,000 American children** 14 years or younger

- **1 in 3** people have intractable/ uncontrolled Epilepsy

- **1 in 26** people in the U.S will be diagnosed with epilepsy sometime during their lifetime.

- **1 in 10** people worldwide will have a seizure during their lifetime.

Common Causes of Epilepsy

- In **6 of 10 people** with Epilepsy the cause is unknown

- For others, *Common Causes* include:

  Brain malformations

  Inborn errors of metabolism

  Fever (febrile seizures)

  Infections of the brain

  Brain injury at birth

  Genetic factors

  Trauma

  Abnormal brain development

  Stroke

Seizure Types

Focal Onset Aware Seizures

- Focal Onset Aware now replaces the term "Simple Partial"

- Involve only one area of the brain

- Person is aware and alert during seizure

- Health symptoms or problems, such as nausea or pain from stomach disorders or tingling and numbness from a pinched nerve, can be mistaken for focal seizures.

- Hallucinations (smells, tastes, sounds, visions) can accompany psychiatric illness or the use of certain drugs.

- Some symptoms (such as déja vu) are experienced by almost everyone at some time.

- Temporary numbness or weakness in a limb or the face sometimes occurs from a transient ischemic attack (TIA), which can be a serious warning sign for a future stroke.

- Migraines, with or without a significant headache, can produce visual, tingling, or other symptoms that can be confused with a seizure.

- Length: Usually seconds to less than 2 minutes

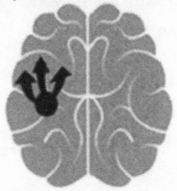

Focal Onset Impaired Awareness Seizures

- Focal Onset Impaired Awareness now replaces the term "Complex Partial"
- Involve only one area of the brain
- These seizures usually start in one area or group of brain cells, most often in the temporal lobe or frontal lobe of the brain. They can also start in other areas too.
- The seizures starting in the frontal lobe tend to be shorter than the ones from the temporal lobe.
- Focal seizures can include involuntary movements called automatisms (aw-TOM-ah-TIZ-ums) like rubbing of the hands, lip-smacking, chewing movements. When they involve the frontal lobes, you may see bicycling movements of the legs or pelvic thrusting or other complex movements.
- Some focal onset impaired awareness seizures (usually ones beginning in the temporal lobe) start with a focal aware seizure (previously call simple partial seizure), which is commonly called an aura.
    - o In this case, the focal aware seizure quickly involves other areas of the brain that affect alertness and awareness.
    - o The person loses awareness and stares blankly. So even though their eyes are open, and they may make movements that seem to have a purpose, in reality "nobody's home."
    - o If the symptoms are subtle, other people may think the person is just daydreaming.
    - o Awareness may be only partially impaired, rather than absent. Any decrease in awareness of the self or environment at any time during a seizure makes it a focal impaired awareness seizure.

- A person's ability to respond may be impaired. Some seizures make the person unable to move yet still aware of what is happening around them.
- Impairment of awareness is similar to the concept of impairment of consciousness.

- Some focal impaired awareness (complex partial) seizures can spread to both sides of the brain. Previously called secondarily generalized seizures, the new name for this is focal to bilateral tonic-clonic seizures.

  - They usually last between 30 seconds and 3 minutes.
  - Afterward, the person may be tired or confused for about 15 minutes and may not be return to normal function for hours.

- **Length of Focal Onset Impaired Awareness Seizure: Up to several minutes**

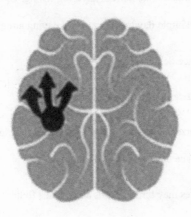

Generalized Onset Absence Seizures

- The older term "Petit Mal" is no longer in use.

- An absence seizure is a generalized onset seizure, which means it begins in both sides of the brain at the same time.

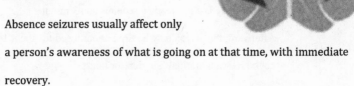

- Absence seizures usually affect only a person's awareness of what is going on at that time, with immediate recovery.

- There are two types of absence seizures that may look a bit different. Both types of seizures are short, and people often don't notice them at first. They may come and go so quickly that no one notices anything wrong. Or observers may mistake the symptoms for simple daydreaming or not paying attention.

- Typical Absence Seizures:

  o These seizures are the most common.

  o The person suddenly stops all activity. It may look like he or she is staring off into space or just has a blank look.

  o The eyes may turn upwards and eyelids flutter.

  o Typical Absence seizures usually last less than 10 seconds.

- Atypical Absence Seizures

  - o These absence seizures are called atypical because they may be longer, have a slower onset and offset, and involve different symptoms.

  - o The seizure still starts with staring into space, usually with a blank look.

  - o There is usually a change in muscle tone and movement. You may see

  - o Blinking over and over that may look like fluttering of the eyelids

  - o Smacking the lips or chewing movements

  - o Rubbing fingers together or making other hand motions

  - o An Atypical absence seizure lasts longer, up to 20 seconds or more.

Generalized Tonic Clonic Seizures

- This type of seizure (also called a convulsion) is what most people think of when they hear the word "seizure." An older term for this type of seizure is "grand mal."

- As implied by the name, they combine the characteristics of tonic and clonic seizures. Tonic means stiffening, and clonic means rhythmical jerking.

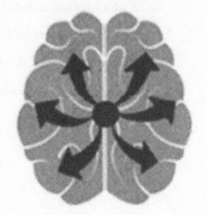

- The tonic phase comes first.

  - o All the muscles stiffen.

  - o Air being forced past the vocal cords causes a cry or groan.

- o The person loses consciousness and falls to the floor.
- o A person may bite their tongue or inside of their cheek. If this happens, saliva may look a bit bloody.
- · After the tonic phase comes the clonic phase.
  - o The arms and usually the legs begin to jerk rapidly and rhythmically, bending and relaxing at the elbows, hips, and knees.
  - o After a few minutes, the jerking slows and stops.
- · The person's face may look dusky or a bit blue if they are having trouble breathing or the seizure lasts too long.
- · The person may lose control of their bladder or bowel as the body relaxes.
- · Consciousness, or a person's awareness, returns slowly.
- · These seizures generally last 1 to 3 minutes. Afterwards, the person may be sleepy, confused, irritable, or depressed.
- · A tonic-clonic seizure that lasts longer than 5 minutes needs immediate medical help. Call 911 for emergency help.
- · A seizure that lasts more than 10 minutes, or three seizures in a row without the person coming to between them, is a dangerous condition. This is called Status Epilepticus; emergency treatment in a hospital is needed.
  - · Length: Usually 1-3 minutes.

Intractable Seizures

- Also referred to as refractory, drug resistant, or uncontrolled seizures

- Only 5% of people (1 out of 20) with intractable Epilepsy get better each year.

- Intractable Epilepsy occurs when a person has failed to become (and stay) seizure free with adequate trials of two Anti-Epileptic Drugs (AEDs)

- These seizure medications must have been chosen appropriately for the person's seizure type, tolerated by the person, and tried alone or together with other seizure medications.

- Non-drug therapies, such as Epilepsy surgery, vagus nerve stimulation, responsive neurostimulation, deep brain stimulation, dietary therapies, or experimental clinical trials, may be good options for some people.

- Most Epilepsy specialists agree that Intractable Epilepsy is Epilepsy for which seizures are frequent and severe enough, or the required therapy for them troublesome enough, to seriously interfere with quality of life.

- Four broad reasons for Intractable Epilepsy:

1. The diagnosis is wrong

2. The treatment is wrong

3. Despite the best treatment, triggers or lifestyle factors may affect seizure control

4. Accurately diagnosed seizures do not respond to the best medical treatment

Status Epilepticus

· *Definition:* A prolonged seizure lasting longer than five minutes or multiple
seizures occurring back-to-back, without full recovery of consciousness in
between.

Convulsive Status Epilepticus:

· The more common form of emergency situation that can occur with prolonged
or repeated tonic-clonic (also called convulsive or grand mal) seizures. Most
tonic-clonic seizures end normally in 1 to 2 minutes, but they may have post-
ictal (or after-effects) symptoms for much longer. This makes it hard to
tell when a seizure begins and ends.

· This type of status epilepticus requires emergency treatment by trained medical
personnel in a hospital setting. This situation can be life-threatening and getting
treatment started fast is vital to lessen the chance of serious complications.

· Oxygen and other support for breathing, intravenous fluids (fluid given into a
blood vessel), and emergency medications are needed.

· At times, medicines called anesthetics are used in the hospital to put a person into
a coma to stop the seizures. Continuous EEG (electroencephalogram)
monitoring may be needed to monitor the seizures and how a person responds to
treatment.

· Tests may also be needed to find the cause of the seizure emergency so it can be tumor, or stroke, may have a worse outlook than those with no other medical problems or known cause.

Non-Convulsive Status Epilepticus:

- This term is used to describe long or repeated focal impaired awareness (complex partial) or absence seizures.

- When Nonconvulsive Status Epilepticus occurs or is suspected, emergency medical treatment in a hospital setting is needed. EEG testing may be needed to confirm the diagnosis first.

- The person may be confused or not fully aware of what is going on, but they are not "unconscious," like in a tonic-clonic seizure.

- These situations can be harder to recognize than convulsive seizures. Symptoms are more subtle and it's hard to tell seizure symptoms from the recovery period.

- There is no consistent timeframe on when these seizures are called an emergency. It depends in part on how long a person's typical seizures are and how often they occur.

- People with this type of status are also at risk for Convulsive Status Epilepticus, thus quick treatment is required.

SUDEP

- SUDEP is the Sudden Unexpected Death of someone in Epilepsy, who was otherwise healthy.

- In SUDEP cases, no other cause of death is found when an autopsy is done.

- Each year, 1 in 1,000 people with Epilepsy die from SUDEP.

- This is the leading cause of death in people with Intractable (uncontrolled) seizures.

- The person with Epilepsy is often found dead, face down, in bed and doesn't appear to have had a convulsive seizure.

- Over one-third of the time, there is a witnessed seizure or signs of a recent seizure close to the time of death.

- Some researchers think that a seizure causes an irregular heart rhythm.

- Other research has shown that breathing difficulties following a seizure lead to death.

~ Background Information used with the permission from *Epilepsy Foundation of America* ~

Learn more at *www.epilepsy.com*

I

. . . . .

A NORMAL DAY - JULY 2010

Middle school had just ended. I had spent the last twelve years, pre-kindergarten through eighth grade, in a small private Christian school. I grew up about sixty miles east of Los Angeles in a small Southern California city. After spending so many years at a small private school, I was preparing myself for the reality of finally going to one of the local public high schools. I knew it would be different, the way the kids spoke, dressed, acted, the music they listened to. I was excited and nervous all at the same time though. I was even more excited for choir, as I had contacted the choir director prior to starting, to see if I could sing in the choir at the high school. I would also be on the football and wrestling teams, which I was not too excited about, but figured I would make plenty of friends and be "cool".

I remember that day in July like it was yesterday, although I cannot give you the exact

3

day only the month. My family, which included my two sisters, my parents, and myself, were all bored at home on that warm summer day. Both of my sisters were in their bedrooms, my father downstairs watching television, my mother watching television in the loft we had, which faced our staircase, and I was in my bedroom watching television as well. All of us tried to stay cool and entertain our boredom.

I finally came out of my bedroom and when I arrived at the top of our staircase about to head down the stairs, I heard a voice. My mother asked me something, "Can you bring me a snack on your way back up?". I stood there, silent, at the top of the staircase for a while. I did not look like my normal self. My mother got concerned, and repeatedly asked, " Are you okay son?" without a response from me for a while. When I finally responded, I told her I was fine. I asked her why she kept asking me that. She told me I had been standing there at the top of the stairs and staring at the staircase for a long time. I replied "I feel fine, I've only been standing here for a couple of seconds. And I already said I'd get your snack!" So, I brushed it off and continued down the stairs to the kitchen.

The fact was, I had not noticed that I had been standing there for as long as I thought I had been. Within a few minutes I got very tired. In fact, so tired that I forgot what my mother asked me to get her, so she came downstairs to get it herself and stayed downstairs with my father and explained to him what she had witnessed about me.

Before I went back upstairs, she asked me again, "Are you sure you feel okay son?"

I replied, "Yeah, I feel fine." But the truth was, I was extremely tired, but an exhausted tired. I ended up going to our loft and falling asleep for a few hours or so. When I woke up from my nap though, things felt different. As if everything had changed instantaneously.

I got worried and panicked, so I went downstairs. My mother was able to tell immediately because there was a worried look on my face. "I don't feel very good, can we go to the Urgent Care please?" I asked her. She agreed to take me. Our Urgent Care was partnered with a small medical group that was local within our area. When we arrived, my mother filled out the tiny slip of paper that was required every time we went. She described what had happened. She then had it time stamped by a tiny machine and dropped it into a slit in the wall so the nurse could call us when they were ready. The room was small, and busy, as it always was. It was not long, probably ten minutes when I heard my name called by the nurse. My mother and I hurried to the door and went in, where they weighed me, took my blood pressure, and the usual. The nurse continued to ask why we were there, and my mother explained the event from earlier that day at the staircase. Without hesitation, the nurse told my mother and myself it sounded like I may have had an episode or seizure, so we should consider going to the Emergency Room if it truly was a seizure. The nurse recommended two hospital Emergency Rooms, we could use the local community one or the *Medical Center* a few miles farther.

We tried the local one, but they were extremely busy, so we ended up at the *Medical Center* a few miles farther. As soon as we checked in, I stood there not knowing what to do, I only heard my mother and the lady going back and forth about what had happened earlier. It all

felt strange, me, a 14-year-old, standing in the middle of an Emergency Room. I then heard what

sounded like them saying I needed to be seen by a physician because it sounded like some

sort of episode or seizure. As my mother and I waited in the Emergency Room to be seen,

worried about what was to come, not really knowing that a longer road was ahead for me, we

heard my name called next. The doctor, I couldn't tell you his name, walked us to a room where

he tested my eyesight, reflexes, strength, all the normal things. Again, my mother told him the

story from earlier, probably tired of telling it. All I remember hearing from that night was in fact,

it was an episode and seizure.

We left and drove home not knowing what to think. When we got home, my mother

explained everything the doctor had told us to my father. Since our small medical group had an

adult neurology department, that was where our insurance had placed me. So, my parents and I

were stuck with our small medical group not knowing how their adult neurology department

would mess me up with wrong medications because they wouldn't know how to treat pediatric

neurology patients. So, now there we were, not knowing how to move forward.

By the time I saw a neurologist from the small medical group, without asking us

questions, or anything about the situation, the neurologist diagnosed me with Epilepsy, which

was technically correct. But, without hesitation he started to prescribe me random medications.

He never actually asked me how I felt at my appointments, and most of the time it had made me drowsy, agitated, and hard to concentrate. It was a new way of life for me. All of it was new to my family, all the while my parents frustrated and constantly fighting with the adult neurologist, trying to get him to understand what the medications were doing to me.

One day our close family friend Martha, who was one of my mother's best friends, recommended a pediatric neurology specialist in Epilepsy. My mother and Martha had known each other for as long as I can remember, long before I was even born. She had seen me grow up, bathed me when I was little, my mother did the same with her daughter. After Martha and my parents talked about the specialist, it was no surprise that it was with the *Medical Center* that we had originally went to the Emergency Room at. I later found out in my college years; they were a part of the National Association of Epilepsy Centers (NAEC) and a level four center. Martha knew of the pediatric neurology because one of her relatives had surgery at that same *Medical Center*, however in a different department, so she constantly gave back to that *Medical Center*.

Unlike the small medical group, I was with, that was the chance to get the right medical help. Martha helped just by recommending us to them and even a specific pediatric neurologist. My parents had received a referral from the *Medical Center* by that time but were now up against the insurance company who wanted to save money and keep me with the small medical group. I was still on the medication prescribed from the adult neurologist and tried to go about my days living life to the best of my ability as my parents fought for me to see a new neurologist.

HIGH SCHOOL BEGINS

TUESDAY, AUGUST 12, 2010

FRESHMAN YEAR had begun at the high school. It was a brand-new school for me. A *public* school to make it more stressful, where I knew absolutely no one. I was nervous, anxious, and even more stressed out than usual. I knew my parents were nervous too, especially with my health condition taking on a whole new level for me. We were still trying to get into the *Medical Center*, so my parents were trying to figure out how they would get me in. At the rate I was headed, I was having two, almost three seizures per day. Even on the medication the adult neurologist was giving me, it was not helping me, or so it seemed. But he was the professional, so we followed his instructions and I kept taking it. My parents had made sure I was well prepared for the school year and contacted the health office to let them know of my condition. They gave them extra medication in case I would need it for any reason.

On the first day of classes, it was busy on campus, and there were many people walking around. Coming from such a small private school my old school had maybe one hundred students or a little more at most. There were thousands of students walking around, I couldn't believe it! It was exciting and stressful trying to find my classes, luckily the buildings all had a letter followed by room numbers. I came to my first class, *Geography*. I sat through it like the rest of the students, read the syllabus, watched other students talk to each other as most knew each other from the public middle schools.

The bell finally rang, and everyone ran out. I slowly walked to the teacher, she was a short lady, I asked if I could talk to her. "Hi, I'm James, but everyone calls me Jimmy."

"Hi Jimmy, what can I do for you?" she asked.

I proceeded to tell her about my health.

"I wanted to let you know I have Epilepsy." I told her.

She didn't seem to mind. Our conversation was short when I realized I was going to be late. She ended up writing me a hall pass to excuse my tardiness to my next class. I hurried along trying to find my second period classroom. It was choir. I tried not to look bad, especially for that class, and in front of Miss Evans, the choir director.

I finally found the performing arts building; it was tucked away in a corner of the campus where no one could really find it. I walked into the classroom, handed a tall, amazon looking lady my hall pass. *Could this be Miss Evans? She looked nothing like what I thought she would.*

HOPE WITHIN ME

"I'm sorry for being late, I couldn't find the building" I told her

"It's okay sweetheart, no one can find this building on their first day" she replied

She seemed so sweet and kind, yet so tall and Amazonian-like. Throughout choir that day, she told us what kind of choir it was and what we would be doing throughout the school year. It was a men's choir. I had never been in a men's choir so it would be interesting to see what kind of songs we would be singing and performing. She also told us how she would use that year and class to see which men she wanted in her *Advanced Mixed Ensemble* the next year, which was the highest of all the choirs at the school. That made me super excited.

With classes only being a certain time length, the bell rang, and once again I waited for all the students to leave. I wanted to tell Miss Evans about my health. I felt it was best to tell all of my teachers. But she had already headed to her office, so I followed her, knocked on her office door and waited. She opened the door and a fragrance of candles rushed out and filled my nostrils and lungs. It was the most delightful smell I had smelled.

"Hello Miss Evans, I just wanted to talk to you about my health really quick." I told her

"Hi Jimmy, you can have a seat here in my office sweetheart." She replied.

I sat on a big, cushioned chair; it was the most comfortable chair I had ever sat in.

"What would you like to talk to me about sweetheart?" Miss Evans asked.

I noticed she said sweetheart a lot, even during class time.

"I have Epilepsy, I was just diagnosed a month ago." I told her

11

She continued by letting me know how I could always go to her if I needed anything. Water, a snack, or to sit down during rehearsal. In that moment I felt safe in her office, in her classroom I knew it would be like no other. The warning bell had rung, so I said thank you and told her I would see her the next day and went on with my day and to the rest of my classes.

It was the end of the school day, and I was glad to be home. My parents had asked me how my first day went and if it all went okay. I told them, like any other kid or teenager, that it went "fine". I was tired, and the only real homework I had that night was to sign all the syllabuses to turn in the next day. I was ready for bed and see what the next day and year would bring me. My parents also had their own homework. They were still trying to convince the insurance how bad the adult neurologist was for me and how the pediatric specialist would be a better fit for a 14-year-old child.

. . . . . .

August went by and I was still having seizures. One, two, and three on some days. The medication barely helped me. The only thing that brought joy to my days was choir at the high school. By the end of August, I had started football. I really hated football if I was to be honest. I only did football to stay somewhat active and to keep my father happy. Although most practices, and all the games, I stood on the sidelines. I think the coaches were afraid to put me in the games because of my Epilepsy.

HOPE WITHIN ME

To my surprise, and by a blessing of God, I came home one day after school and found out my referral had finally accepted by our insurance so I could go see the pediatric Epilepsy neurologist at the *Medical Center*. Since I was having so many seizures throughout the day, without any improvement with the medication, the referral was approved. I would finally get a new neurologist!

By the end of August and early September I was in the groove of things academically. I had a new pediatric neurologist, Doctor Michaels, who had officially diagnosed me with Complex Partial Seizures (now called Focal Onset Impaired Awareness Seizures) not just general Epilepsy. So, I was no longer on my old medication, I would be prescribed what was called *Levetiracetam*, and I started taking that.

It was a September morning, and I was late for my first period class at school because my ride had showed up late. So, when I went to my first class the door was locked. I knocked but no one answered. I stood there for a minute before I realized that we were supposed to meet in the media center on campus to work on our papers. When I finally realized that, I took a few steps about to head to the media center before I froze in the center of the hallway. I felt a funny feeling in me. After the funny feeling was gone, I felt something weird on my shorts, so I looked down and my shorts were wet. I felt them and thought my water had leaked from my backpack I was wearing, but everything was dry inside my bag. I rushed to the nearest bathroom and patted my shorts trying to figure out why they were wet, when suddenly I started to get tired. I realized at that moment I had a seizure and that I had urinated on myself. I sat in a bathroom stall and cried. Not only did I have a seizure standing up in the middle of the hallway, with other late students walking past me, watching, but I had also urinated on myself.

I realized five minutes later I needed to get to first period still. So, I got up and used the hand dryer machine to dry my shorts. Once they were dry, I walked to the media center and sat down to work on my paper. I went about my day, and all I could think about throughout the day was what had happened that morning in the hallway. When I got home, I told my parents what happened. My mother broke down crying, and my father logged the seizure. We were to log all of my seizure activity and describe them with Doctor Michaels at my neurology appointments, which were approximately every two to three months.

THE FOOTBALL GAME - OCTOBER 2010

In October of 2010, an old friend Cristine, who went to the same private Christian school with me when I was younger ended up going to the same high school as me. Cristine and I were close at the private school since we were the only people with anything in common there and also having been the only people of color there, me being Mexican and her being African American. Since I was on the freshman football team, and no one really knew who I was, we both decided it would be fun to go to our first varsity football game together. It was probably five or six o'clock when my mother dropped both of us off. We found a spot a little over mid-way up in the bleachers to watch the game. We never realized that most people at these games were only really here to socialize. However, we got to halftime and we both decided we would go to the snack bar. So, we both went down there and luckily beat the line and were able to come back up fast. We sat there and laughed at the marching band and talked a while before I realized I had to use the bathroom.

"I'll be right back; I need to use the bathroom."

"Okay, hurry up though, I think it's going to start again." Cristine semi yelled.

I hurried down the bleachers to the bathrooms and by the time I finished washing my hands I heard the buzzer, ready for the second half.

I rushed through the people who tried to get their snacks. I reached the bottom of the bleachers, about to make my ascent up when I suddenly felt that funny feeling. Ignoring it, I made my way up the bleachers, until I fell. My friend Cristine eyed me and noticed something wasn't right the second I stopped mid-way from the bottom. People walked past me, and even stepped over me. She ran down to me, pushing people out of the way. By the time I came out of my seizure, Cristine described to me what happened. We sat through the rest of the game, still enjoying it, and laughing. When my mother picked us up after the game, Cristine described what had happened. My mother was furious, not at me, but at the people at the game. Cristine had told her how no one had helped her or me. They all walked over me, stared, and left me on the ground. To this day, I don't blame anyone at the game, who could have known. A helping hand would have been nice, but all I was left with was a good friend, Cristine, and a memory that was logged into my seizure journal.

MAGNETIC RESONANCE IMAGING - NOVEMBER 2011

It was the middle of November and my second appointment with Doctor Michaels arrived. Since my last appointment, we described and showed him the journal we kept with all the seizures I had. Especially the two major ones where I urinated on myself and was alone and the other when I was with my friend at the football game. Doctor Michaels decided two things, the first was to increase my *Levetiracetam* and the second was that I needed an MRI (Magnetic Resonance Imaging) scan of my brain. I will never forget how he explained what an MRI was and how they went about it for their pediatric neurological patients.

"So, we will lay you down on your back, and put a cage over your head so that you don't move it at all because you have to be completely still."

The minute he said "put a cage over your head" that made me nervous, but I continued to

JAMES VALENCIA

listen.

"Then, we will give you a blanket, so you don't get cold, and we will put you in this giant tube that acts like a giant magnet. You will be in there for approximately thirty to forty-five minutes. It will take pictures of your brain so I can look at them later."

Doctor Michaels explained all of this to my father and myself. I think both of us looked a little confused and not knowing what to think as this was the first *real* test I've ever had scheduled. At the end of the appointment, we all smiled, my father and I thanked Doctor Michaels, shook his hand, and went on our way.

The MRI was scheduled for the following week. All I remember about that day was walking into the room and having them ask me to empty my pockets. In front of me was a giant machine that looked like a tube with a skinny bed that slid out. The technician led me to a bed and had me lay flat on my back. He asked me to lay my arms at my side then brought a warm blanket. He put it over me and told me to pull my arms out and put them down again. He then gave me a little button attached to a cord. He instructed that if at any time I needed to get out of the machine to push the button and they would let me out. Whether it was anxiety, claustrophobia, even if I felt like I was about to have a seizure, to push it. After he gave me all of the instructions, he put the cage over my face which kept my face from moving from side to side. He then pushed me into the machine which made me feel small, but I knew the test needed to be done, so I stayed as still as I could and closed my eyes. Suddenly, I heard and even felt a giant noise around me. *The magnets* I thought to myself. They were loud, and I felt them going around

me too. I was given disposable ear plugs at the beginning of the session, but I felt like they didn't

help much. I laid there, inside a giant machine, wondering what Doctor Michaels would find or

figure out after all of that, and how I got to be there in the first place.

"Alright, that's it." A faint voice said.

I felt the bed move again. I opened my eyes, and within seconds I saw the light of the

room again. The technician lifted the cage off my head.

"That was forty-five minutes?" I asked.

"Yup." He said

It all felt so fast, so surreal. He led me to my belongings I had taken out of my pockets

earlier and then he led me to the door back to my parents who sat right outside and waited for

me. We went home, and I couldn't be more excited to be home.

. . . . .

It neared the holiday season, and Christmas was my favorite time of the year. The

holidays came and went that year. I had a couple of seizures here and there, logged them in the

journal we kept. My parents and I had to patiently wait for the January appointment with Dr.

Michaels at that point.

ELECTROENCEPHALOGRAM

JANUARY 2011. My Freshman year of high school still and it was time for me to finally have another appointment with Doctor Michaels again. My parents and I still wondered what he had found, if anything, from the MRI Scan. To our surprise, my MRI Scan came back normal. No abnormalities, which in essence was a good thing, but we wanted to know more. So, Doctor Michaels wanted to do something that some pediatric and adult neurology specialists do. He was going to schedule me for a Video EEG (Electroencephalogram). He explained to us what an EEG was first.

A normal EEG watched the electrical activity on the different areas of the brain, and if there were any abnormalities it would catch it because it would be recording it on a computer. A Video EEG involved being video recorded while having a normal EEG. So, if a person, say someone with Epilepsy, has a seizure they would know where on the brain the seizure is occurring, and the video would show what the person is doing and looked like at the time of the event. Doctor Michaels explained how it needed to be done in the hospital, so I would need to be hospitalized for five to seven days. He scheduled it within two weeks, which gave my parents and myself time to inform school administration of the situation and my teachers so I could get homework ahead of time.

VIDEO ELECTROENCEPHALOGRAM

SATURDAY, JANUARY 29, 2011

It was almost time for my Video EEG. My family and I were almost ready to check into the children's section of the *Medical Center*. They took us up to the fourth floor, as that's where pediatric neurology was at, and brought us into a room. We set all my things down. I had brought all my homework my teachers gave me for the upcoming week. Staying only in my boxers, I changed into a hospital gown and laid down on the uncomfortable bed, which unfortunately would be mine for next week. The technician for the EEG came in after I finished changing and applied the wires to my head. The technician pulled out a box full of tiny wires and some type of glue that smelled weird. I let him do his thing. The wires were placed in different spots on my head. Once they were placed on my head, white bandaging was wrapped around the entire top of my head so the wires weren't exposed or couldn't move. By the end, I had a big, thick cord that stuck out of the top of my head that led to the wall that gave it all power and sent signals to the technician and neurologist as it recorded data 24/7.

As soon as the wires were attached, the technician handed me a button and left. Doctor Michaels arrived shortly after. He greeted my family and me with a big, friendly smile like always, and sat with us, commented on a great job the technician did on wrapping the wires, and then explained how the process of the week would go.

"So, James" He spoke to me, "feel free to do any homework or reading of course."

Because that was the one thing I wanted to do while being propped up inside of a hospital, was learn geometry and read fifty pages for English class. That's all I could think.

"Mom, Dad, and James of course, as you are aware, we are here to do a Video EEG with James." Doctor Michaels continued, "The point of this is for James to *actually have a seizure.*"

My ears propped up at that.

"We are going to do a series of things to try to do that."

He explained to us.

" We will start with sleep deprivation, which we will begin tonight. Then move to hyperventilation and flashing lights, with his eyes closed of course, in the coming days. Next, we will start to slowly decrease his medication. All of this *should* lead to a seizure. We will be monitoring this 24/7, as I have direct access to it from my office. So, we will know if there is any electrical activity."

HOPE WITHIN ME

He spoke to me, "James, if you feel like you are about to have or having a seizure, push that button. It marks it in the recorder."

Doctor Michael's words worried all us, but we knew we should trust him.

Eventually, it was time for my parents to go home, as visiting hours had ended. They promised they would be back the next day, so as we said goodnight to each other, I knew I'd see them the next day. After they left, the night nurse came in and told me I had to stay awake until one or two o 'clock in the morning.

The first thing Doctor Michaels wanted to try was sleep deprivation. The one thing I can tell you about that hospitalization was that we tried it all. The days went by slowly. First, we tried sleep deprivation, then hyperventilation, and flashing lights. At that point we were three days in, and still no seizure activity. *Everything appeared normal! How though? I had been having so many on a regular basis, and in the hospital nothing.* The first few days had been nice though, other than the occasional visits from Doctor Michaels who gave updates on the next strategy. I had visits from my aunts and uncles, and my sisters who came with my parents sometimes. My grandparents came a few times which made me happy. I laugh at it now, but my grandfather brought me two cheeseburgers and fries one day because he told me, "you don't need to just eat that nasty hospital food mijo.".

With only a few more days left to actually *have* a seizure, the strategy was simple, start tapering off the medication and sleep deprive me like crazy. Everyday Doctor Michaels came in and told us how everything looked normal. Again, we tried hyperventilation and flashing lights one more time...nothing happened. It was the weirdest thing to him, my family and me. We all wanted answers. At one point, my medication was tapered so low, I was off of it completely by my last night. There was still no seizure activity at all. Finally, the hospital had told my parents that they were getting ready to discharge me. My six days, which is what the referral was for, was over. The morning of discharge, they started me back on my normal medication dosage again. My parents weren't at the *Medical Center* yet, but my discharge papers were in the works. It all happened so fast that morning, and all I remember was I felt a funny feeling and it finally happened.

The nurse and the Video EEG technician walked into the room and noticed the button in my hand. I hadn't even noticed I pushed it. My parents were on their way up when they were told, and Doctor Michaels was headed up too. It was the first time having a seizure was a good thing. I was tired though, like most of my seizures made me. Luckily, I was headed home that day. So, my parents got the car ready and the discharge papers. We were headed home. It had been a long week for me, sitting and doing homework in a hospital bed all week with my father who went back and forth to the school turning it in for me. Most of all, the loneliness I felt in the hospital when there was no one there, crushed me like no other, but I knew that there was good that came and would come from it. It took all six days of the week, but still, a light of faith shined through on that last day, Friday February 4, 2011.

HOPE WITHIN ME

. . . . . .

Since my Video EEG, going back to school made me happy. Singing in choir and the interaction with other students had felt good. Miss Evans and the *Advanced Mixed Ensemble* gave me a card, which was nice. It was filled with many great compliments about me and my voice with sincere 'get wells'. Choir became my 'home-away-from-home' at school, and I couldn't have been happier that spring.

In March of 2011, I had my follow up appointment with Doctor Michaels. My parents and I went and met with him. He wanted to discuss what he had seen and found in the Video EEG. What he had discovered was that the seizure I had, right before I was discharged from the hospital, came from what seemed like one of my temporal lobes. But the images and recordings had been blurred together. So, what he wanted to do, to see if it would help, was to add another medication on top of my *Levetiracetam*. He prescribed me *Oxcarbazepine*, which I was to take one 600mg tablet/2x daily on top of the regular *Levetiracetam*.

The memory that haunted me the most from that visit was what I was shown next. He pulled the video from the EEG and asked if I wanted to see it. I did want to see it, but I was also too nervous to say no. He played the part where I had my seizure. He pointed out every detail. I saw my father stare at the screen, analyzing it. My mother's eyes teared up. And for the first time I watched what I looked like having a Focal Impaired Awareness Seizure.

JAMES VALENCIA

"The glazed eyes, drooling, clenching your fingers" Doctor Michaels described to me

"It's different watching it isn't it?" He asked me.

"Yeah." I replied. Barely able to speak as my own eyes had started to water like my

mother's. I wanted to breakdown and cry at how terrifying and helpless I looked in the video.

It was real. The first time I'd ever seen myself have a seizure, especially on video. On

the ride home, I remember talking to my mother about it and how hard it was to watch it, and she

just nodded, as she wiped tears as they fell. My father with a stern face like always. In my head

though, I was about to get a new medication, with a hope that was the answer and was going to

help lessen all of our problems...*my* problems.

HIGH SCHOOL CHOIR AUDITION - MAY 2011

As the academic year came to an end that year, and freshman year and my first official year in a public school was almost over, I had gotten ready for choir auditions. Miss Evans had made a real liking to me since I had arrived at the high school, and even more so, to my voice. She constantly told the upperclassmen about my voice. Every so often there were a group of upper-class girls or boys in our men's choir class to listen to us. It seemed like they were only there when we sang music I had a solo in, which I felt like Miss Evans told them we would be rehearsing that day. This put more pressure on me to do great at the audition for the advanced mixed group. I knew she rarely let any sophomore students in that group.

It was more pressure to be in the advanced choir because there were rumors of a possible traveling opportunity, either to Europe or New York. It all came from the upperclassmen, who had no real source they could give anyone. Miss Evans had mentioned nothing of the sort that spring. There were just performances and rehearsals. There were a select few that were close to Miss Evans, I was one of them who she eventually let sit in her office when she would go out to lunch. We would hang out, talk, and sit in her chairs and even at her office desk. She really trusted us, even with her keys at times. What we really wanted to know was if we were traveling anywhere the following year. Still, Miss Evans never mentioned anything all of that spring.

During the week of auditions, Miss Evans used the men's choir class time to audition us boys. I went somewhere in the middle of all the boys in our class. She made me sing some scales on neutral syllables, tested my tonal memory, made me sight read, the normal music stuff. At the end of my test, she told me the list would be posted later during the week and not to worry.

Everyone flocked to the bulletin board that Friday afternoon . There were only thirty spots total, which meant six or eight tenor spots. I waited out the crowd, and when it cleared, I went to look. I sifted through the tenor two names. I wasn't there. Next, I sifted through the tenor one names. There I was! And to my surprise I was the only sophomore boy. I looked through all of the soprano and alto names, and only one sophomore girl made it, and I didn't know her. Incredible, out of the thirty something students, two sophomores made the *Advanced Mixed Ensemble*. Sophomore year hadn't even started, and it was off to a good start.

HOPE WITHIN ME

. . . . .

It was the end of July that year, when my parents received an email from Miss Evans. She had sent it to all of the members of the *Advanced Mixed Ensemble*. I remember asking my parents what the email was about, and they told me that Miss Evans was debating on taking the choir on a tour in the spring of 2012. The options were Europe or New York and Carnegie Hall. It stated that on "back to school night" the parents were going to vote on where they would like the students to go, based on price. Of course, I wanted the Europe option, but I was fine with the New York option too.

In my head though, I remembered all the talk from the previous year and the rumors in the choirs. The upperclassmen had been right all along. I was excited for sophomore year to start in the fall so my parents were able to vote for one of the places for me to travel. I thought to myself that one of those trips was going to be the highlight of my sophomore year.

AUGUST 2011

SOPHOMORE YEAR was in full force as the academic year had begun at the high school. I was placed in the advanced mixed choir at the end of my freshman year, so things were off to a great start. The night of "back to school night", Miss Evans let the students come with their parents and sit on the choir risers in the back while the parents sat up front in chairs to vote on the trip. The choir members thought we would get the answer that night, instead the answer wouldn't come until the next day. Most of us in the choir wanted Europe, but when we sat through "back to school night" with our parents and heard Europe's $7,000 compared to New York's $4,000 we all knew the parents would choose New York. Part of me was fine with that. I was okay with any traveling. Miss Evans told everyone in the room that she would email the parents the next day. So, as I arrived home after school the next day, I waited for the news and the answer, already knowing what it was. My parents told me what it was...New York and Carnegie Hall. I was excited beyond my wildest dreams. I would be singing in Carnegie Hall! Although we wouldn't get the music until that spring semester, all we knew at that moment was that were going to be singing with other choirs from around the country and with a live orchestra. What else could a 15-year-old sophomore in high school who was passionate about music want?

The only problem my parents and I ran into with the New York trip that year was the price, which was understandable, as most of the students did. There were many fundraising opportunities throughout that fall and spring, but it was still not enough at times as we had installments due on certain weeks. So, I took it upon myself to get creative that year. I took a shoebox, went to the store, and bought candy bars and other candies, put them in the shoebox, hid them, and sold them out of my backpack. I later found out it was completely illegal. However, I made around $20-$40 per week. I was able to pay off over half my New York trip just from the candy out of my backpack.

During my freshman year the men's choir was fun, but it felt better to be in the mixed choir. However, the music Miss Evans chose for the advanced group was hard. Unlike the men's choir, where all the music was mostly English, the *Advanced Mixed Ensemble* sang mostly in

34

different languages like German, Italian, French, and on rare occasions, English. Even with the hard music, being in the advanced choir was fun, especially with all the other students. Everyone in the choir knew about my Epilepsy. I told them the first week of classes, and how they could help me if I ever had a seizure during rehearsal. They were incredibly supportive, which made me happy. I felt at home when I was in that class. We always referred to each other as family. Fall of 2011 was off to a good start. Choir went well, academics I had always kept decent, I was still on the football team (I still stood on the sidelines), and the wrestling team I never worried about because the practices were in the springtime and I was automatically placed on junior varsity. I still had seizures though, but decreased to two or three times a week, which still wasn't good, but better than the previous year. The *Oxcarbazepine* had helped, but slowly.

It was time for my fall appointment with Doctor Michaels. My father and I went to my appointment and brought the seizure journal. We showed him the journal and described anything we could remember from the ones that had happened at home. Since I still had two and three per week, Doctor Michaels decided to change my medication a bit. He took me completely off the *Levetiracetam* and raised my *Oxcarbazepine*. I started to take two 600mg tablets/2x daily instead of the one tablet/2x daily. He told us since the *Levetiracetam* wasn't doing anything, and the *Oxcarbazepine* was helping, it was more beneficial to only take the one medication. So, once again, we shook hands with Doctor Michaels and walked out of his office with my father and went home.

JAMES VALENCIA

. . . .

Football season had ended, and spring of 2012 arrived. I prepared for wrestling practice. Although I still had seizures, the practices weren't hard. I would actually get to practice compared to football where I stood on the sidelines. I soon found out I was able to use my health condition to my advantage during practice and to 'help' my fellow practice mates, though I regret it now looking back on it. During wrestling practices, I went up to the coaches and told them I wouldn't feel good. Or I told them I had a seizure earlier in the day when I actually didn't. Some practices my wrestling partner and me pretended that I had a seizure, so the coach would cancel the rest of practice. It only made it worse on days I actually did have seizures and couldn't go.

As I look back on all of what I did during that time, I would never do that now. Especially on the road Epilepsy would take me on and knowing of what it takes others on too, that is something I would never do beyond my high school years. Having been a 15-year-old and diagnosed a year ago at that time, I wanted to use it.

NEW YORK & CARNEGIE HALL

MARCH 14, 2012

As spring became chaotic with wrestling matches and choir rehearsals, especially with extra

rehearsals for Carnegie Hall in New York City, it soon became time to leave for the big trip. We

flew out of Los Angeles. The flight was five and a half hours to New York and six hours back, as

it's always longer to come back west. We had prepared Mozart's *Te Deum* which was to be

accompanied with a live orchestra! The trip went by faster than expected. Most of the days in the

city we just woke up, got a cheap bagel and coffee off the street vender outside, rehearsed, ate

lunch, rehearsed, walked around the city, slept, repeated the next day. There were only two days

we actually got to go see the city and walk around and sight see. The city was beautiful and

glowed like no other at night! And the night of the performance, Sunday March 18, 2012,

JAMES VALENCIA

Carnegie Hall was amazing, and it resonated, unlike the choir room. On the last day in the city, all of the students spread out to look around one last time before we loaded up the bus and headed to the airport to come back to California. The plane landed on Monday March 19, 2012. Miss Evans and I had spoken about it later and all we could say was how memorable it was. She was nice enough to let me keep the score we learned the music from.

. . . . .

With two months left of the academic year, it seemed to end fast. Though to me, it felt like it had only begun. Wrestling season had ended, some of the matches that year I had won and some I had lost. And there were no more choir music or performances that year. Miss Evans had also put the new choir list up for next year. However, I wasn't surprised when I saw my name under the advanced mixed group. It was most of the same people from the previous year. I was excited for Junior year of high school.

What a year sophomore year had been that year for everyone. Though, we were all glad the academic year had ended.

CHURCH BEACH TRIP - JUNE 2012

I was able to relax from school and doctor appointments. Aside from all of the normal busyness of classes and appointments, I still attended my regular high school youth group at my church, which met on Wednesday nights around six o'clock until eight thirty or nine o'clock. But because it was summertime, the church had moved to their summer sessions where they would go on small outings, trips, and some of the regular things they did during the normal school year. They knew most families travelled during the summer, so they planned ahead of time and sent out flyers with events they had planned. I looked forward to these Wednesday nights and planned events, never as much as choir though. But I still loved how it brought me closer to God. My relationship with God and faith were important to me. The events of youth group and church seemed to make this particular summer go faster than usual though.

It was the end of June and the high school youth group would be getting ready for an event. It was the summer beach trip! I was excited, as I had not been to the beach all summer or year. I looked forward to going with friends from the youth group, some who I went to the old private school with and others who I didn't, and the youth pastor. Some of the boys were my age, and like many at school, knew of my Epilepsy. Once we arrived at the beach, we instinctively ran to the ocean. There's something about the Southern California water that you don't get anywhere else. We dove through the waves and splashed water at each other before we headed back to the sand and tossed a football around. The two boys I was with went to an opposite high school and were also on the football team. We eventually got hungry, and it was time to eat. Everyone roasted their hot dogs on a stick over a giant fire pit, so the three of us did the same, laughing about school stories and what junior year might look like for us.

After we ate, we threw the football around again before we had gotten bored, so we decided to run to the ocean again. I let the two of them swim out as far as they could, which was only to the buoy. The two of them called my name once they were there,

"Jimmy! Jimmy! Come out here!" They both yelled out to me.

I just ignored them and continued to dive through the waves. They headed back my way, which by the grace of God I'm thankful for every day of my life. Right before I went through one of the waves, I stopped. A wave, larger than the one before, was headed toward me, but I had frozen. I felt that funny feeling again. My friends were headed toward me, noticing something wrong. The next thing I knew, water had rushed over my head and I was being pulled out. My two friends had seen me freeze before I went under the large wave of water. They pulled me out to the best of their ability before they flagged down a lifeguard. Once the lifeguard had me, I was dragged onto the sand and laid on my back. When I finally came out of my seizure my youth pastor was there along with my two friends to make sure I was okay. My two friends later explained what had happened, and I later told them I only remembered stopping in front of the wave before I went under it.

My youth pastor, who was no older than twenty-nine at the time, put a beach towel around me and the four of us walked over to the fire pit. It was around six or seven o'clock by that time and everyone had started to roast smores. I tried to enjoy the rest of the evening, so I roasted smores with my two friends who had essentially saved me. Around eight thirty we started to pack everything up to leave for the hour and a half drive back home. I knew my youth pastor, or I, needed to tell my parents what had happened. My youth pastor and me both told them about the incident and how my two friends pulled me up from the water and the lifeguard put me on the sand, but how I still "enjoyed" the rest of the evening.

When I got home that night, my parents asked if I was okay, I told them "yeah". I went straight to my bedroom, closed my door, and cried. It was a silent type of cry, where you cry so hard no one hears. I was angry at myself, at God, at how I was.

JAMES VALENCIA

I hate my life. It's not fair, I never asked for any of this. To just wake up one day and be like this. God, how could you allow this? What did I do to be like this? And in the ocean this time where I could have drowned and died.

Little did I know how that beach trip changed the course of my life as I lived with Epilepsy. Never to put my feet into the ocean again. Where would have been somewhere I once loved to go; I now dreaded. I now only stayed on the sand or made excuses not to go. At swimming pools, only sticking my feet in the shallow end due to constant fear. Bodies of water had started to become a living nightmare.

FALL 2012

JUNIOR YEAR of high school had started, and it felt like every school year kept starting earlier as it was the first week of August again. It was the same routine as the previous years and other classes. The first week was 'get-to-know you' and syllabus week, and the second week was "back to school night".

Being a varsity wrestler was nice junior year, and practices were fun. It made life less complicated, and everyone on campus knew who I was, either for choir or wrestling. I was able to focus on the choir music Miss Evans assigned. Although Junior year was good, I started to notice one thing, everyone had started to get their driver's license. I started to notice it in November. All of my classmates were starting to drive and get cars. I was still unable to drive because of my Epilepsy. I would need to go a whole year without a seizure, but I was still having them. Although the *Oxcarbazepine* had seemed to stabilize and lower my seizure activity, I would still have them once or twice a month. Doctor Michaels would refer to those seizures as break through seizures. As unsettling and frustrating as it was to watch my peers grow and get their learners permit and driver's license, I still kept optimistic I would eventually be seizure free in the near future.

VAGUS NERVE STIMULATION - JANUARY 2013

It was that time again, as it had been a few months already, although it had not felt like it. I would not forget that visit with Doctor Michaels.

"Good morning Dad" He shook my father's hand.

"Good morning James, how are you both doing today?"

He shook my hand then we all sat down in the chairs. My father answered him and explained how I was still having seizures even with the medication.

"Well, it's too soon to try to increase James' medication. Let's see if his body will adjust over the next few months." Doctor Michaels explained.

What he said next took both my father and myself by surprise.

"There is a device called the *VNS (Vagus Nerve Stimulation)*." Doctor Michaels explained to us what it was and printed us the information.

"A brief overview of how it works: the *VNS* or *Vagus Nerve Stimulation* is a device that treats focal (old name: partial) seizures that don't respond to AEDs (Anti-Epileptic Drugs)/ medications. This is known as drug resistant or Intractable Epilepsy. It works by preventing or lessening seizures by sending regular, mild pulses of electrical energy to the brain via the vagus nerve. The device is implanted in the left chest, and a wire is attached to the device and wound around the vagus nerve sending pulses to the nerve. The person is usually not aware it is working. If the person is aware they are having a seizure, they have a magnet they can swipe over the device in their chest and it will activate an extra burst of stimulation to the brain."

Doctor Michaels explained all of this to my father and myself before he moved on to another extreme option that we both knew we didn't want for a teenager.

"So that is one option, if James ever needs it. There is also another option that proves to be successful in some cases that need it. There's surgery."

My father and I just looked at each other for a while before we looked back. "As a last resort, if you are a candidate for surgery, it has proven successful, especially with the upgrades in technology now. However, you will need to be a candidate for both the *VNS* and surgery." Doctor Michaels explained.

"Those are just some newer advances in technology. Let's see how he is doing in a few months with the *Oxcarbazepine* though. I'm confident his body will adjust to the medication ."

HOPE WITHIN ME

As my father and I shook hands with Doctor Michaels and left the office, we knew immediately we weren't sold on either the *VNS* or surgery. I definitely didn't want a device implanted in my chest or my brain cut open.

We had arrived at home to let my mother know everything he had told us. She was interested in both, but my father and I weren't. A 15-year-old having brain surgery just didn't sound right. What about the cognitive development it could harm? None of us really knew, it was more fear than anything. And the *VNS*, I didn't want a device in my chest, it would haunt me. So, there we were, determined to find the right medication for me to live out the best life I could.

CHOIR ELECTIONS - APRIL 2013

It neared the end of the school year again, and it was time for the annual election of officers for the advanced choir. I had not even thought about being an officer, I had never thought I was a leader type of person. That's when Miss Evans asked me to come into her office.

"Jimmy, sweetheart, can you come into my office please?"

I had no idea what she wanted. *Maybe she wanted me to run a pass to the front office?* I thought to myself, as I walked to her office.

"Hi Miss Evans." I said as I walked in and smiled. She shut the door behind me. I took a seat on one of her comfortable chairs.

"Have you considered running for an office for next year?" she asked.

"Not really. I don't think I would be good at leadership." I replied.

"You should consider running for President of *Advanced Mixed Ensemble*." She told me.

I couldn't believe what I heard her tell me. *Me, run for President? Who would vote?*

"I'll consider it. It sounds interesting and fun. I really love this choir."

"You should, there's no one better for the position sweetheart." I left, shocked.

I walked back into the choir room; everyone was talking to each other. It was like we were given the rest of that rehearsal off. The current choir President had walked up to me and asked me if I was okay. I had told her "yeah". She asked me what Miss Evans wanted, so I proceeded to tell her how Miss Evans wanted to know if I was going to run for an office, specifically President. The current President gave a little laugh.

"No one will vote for you; they will vote for her."

She told me as she pointed to another junior girl in the choir.

"Why not?" I asked her.

"Because they won't listen to you. You just don't give off that vibe of authority or leadership."

She chuckled.

"And you *do*, Miss President?" I said sarcastically before I walked away.

She looked surprised I had sassed her. After I walked away, I felt more energy than I had when I was in Miss Evans' office. I was determined at that point to not only run for President, but to be the President. So, I decided to run for the President's position.

HOPE WITHIN ME

It was May, and the day of the election came for choir officers. I had been ready as there was just the junior girl and me who wanted to be the President. We both prepared our speeches. The loser would be Vice President. She was nervous, which in my mind told me that she wouldn't do well under pressure. She finished, so I went up in front of the choir and said what I wrote, but by memory and off script. The choir seemed to enjoy me better. I had made eye contact with the current president, clearly upset at how good I had done. At the end of my speech, Miss Evans went up in front of the choir and talked about both candidates. I noticed she started to defend me more, but I let her. She then sent us both outside to let the current President and Vice President tally the votes. We stood outside for about ten to fifteen minutes. When we were let back into the room again, the two of us were confused because no one spoke. We stared at the choir, then they all pointed to the white board. Written in giant letters were:

PRESIDENT: Jimmy V.

I had felt bad at first because they didn't write Vice President and the junior girl's name up, but it was a given who the Vice President was. Plus, I had won. In the last weeks of that year, once the new choir list was up for the following year, the junior girl and me got over our differences and threw a barbeque for the new advanced choir as a "get-to-know-you". It was so the new choir knew each other before the next academic year. It ended up being a successful junior year in all, despite my health.

Fall 2013

SENIOR YEAR had arrived for me. I was the President of the advanced choir, and what was more exciting was that my cousin Breezy had made it into the advanced choir along with me, as she had made the alto section. I couldn't believe she was a sophomore already. That year was a busy year for me. I would think about college, and what I wanted to do for a career. There was so much to do senior year. Plus, my health had been doing pretty well too. I had gone months at a time without seizures that year. I would go almost two months without a seizure. Doctor Michaels was happy, my parents were happy, and I was somewhat happy. It all seemed as if everything was going to stabilize.

That fall, I heard that my cousin Breezy took voice lessons with Miss Evans, so I decided I was going to start taking lessons that fall too. I felt confident that the path I wanted to go down for my career was choral music. I wanted to inspire students the way she had inspired me. The way she gave me a place to feel safe and at home, I wanted to give that to students of my own one day. So, I started taking voice lessons and learned basic music theory. Miss Evans also started to teach me art songs in German, Italian, and English.

"Do you have any schools or universities you want to apply to?"

she asked me during one of my lessons.

"There's one school. It's a tiny Liberal Arts College not far from here."

I told her.

"Sweetheart, that's my alma mater." She pulled out a picture of her at the school.

The next day at school, she looked up the audition requirements and what I needed to do for auditions. She chose two pieces of vocal music that fit the requirements, a German and Italian piece. We practiced them during my lesson times, and I worked on them at home too.

While I learned the audition pieces, I was also be involved in the regional Honor Choir held in Southern California. I was in the Men's Choir. That didn't take as much work because we were given recordings to learn the music. Throughout October and November, time was spent with the Southern Regional Honor Choir. My cousin Breezy would also be there, in the Women's choir. It all came together on November 23, 2013 for a giant choral concert for the families and the choral performing arts community.

Once Regional Honor Choir was over though, I was back to focusing on college audition music. When my pieces were ready, which took a month for memorization of the German and Italian, Miss Evans had me stand in front of the advanced ensemble and practice speaking the name of the music, composers, and had me sing the pieces. Miss Evans was a pianist who taught choir, so she accompanied me. We did that once or twice a week until I was comfortable in front of people and I felt prepared for my audition in February.

Before Auditions, the first requirement was to apply to the Liberal Arts College and then to the School of Music within it. I applied to both in November. Like any senior in high school, anxious and nervous of results, I waited. I kept rehearsing until the audition in February, to ensure I would be at my best and try to receive an acceptance.

. . . . .

In December, I had another visit with Doctor Michaels. Though there had been breakthrough seizures every two months, the medication was working fairly well. Any higher on the medication and the FDA would likely not allow the dose, as I would be at the maximum dosage for the age and weight. So, we kept the dosage the same, confident my body would adjust with time.

COLLEGE AUDITION DAY

SATURDAY, FEBRUARY 1, 2014

Audition day had arrived. It was a Saturday morning, when my mother and I pulled into the

small Liberal Arts College, not far from my house. It was a small building that read *School of*

Music. I was nervous and eager, not knowing what to expect from the voice panel in the audition

room. I wore black dress pants, a light blue button down, a dark blue striped tie, a black blazer,

and black dress shoes. I felt professional, and eager that day. I walked into the small building and

was greeted by current music students who led me to where I could warm up my voice. I warmed

up a bit, sang through a few spots on my audition music, but not the whole thing. I was then

taken down to the performance hall where I was greeted by a few of the voice faculty members

and the pianist who would play with me during the audition. After the audition, the faculty

members were polite and honest. They weren't harsh or mean like I thought they would be.

I walked out of there with confidence. My mother had picked me up in front of the same building afterwards, and we went to get lunch to take home. A few years later, I found out I was supposed to stay for a theory placement, but I would have been placed in the lowest course anyway, so I know I didn't miss much.

In, Miss Evans decided the *Advanced Mixed Ensemble* was going to perform at a festival at a university about an hour away from the high school. It was during school hours, so everyone was happy. We all left in the afternoon, and when we had arrived, each choir there only had enough time to warm up on the stage and then sit down in their seats before their performance. However, when I went to sit in my seat, I started feeling funny. I remember that day I had made sure to bring all of my medication with me and water, but it wasn't time for it yet. Some of the students from another choir saw me and helped me sit down in my seat along with members of the advanced choir. I felt fine after, I just felt embarrassed. But the students who had helped me sat in front of me and asked if I was okay. It was a nice feeling, that students from another school were kind enough to help me during a seizure. I had noticed Miss Evans was sitting to my right and my cousin Breezy to my left, which was fine because I figured most of the members of the ensemble knew I was close to both of them. I was still disappointed though, another seizure at the end of February. This had meant my seizures were now one month apart.

MARCH 2014

It was time for another appointment with Doctor Michaels in March, and I was scared to tell him

about all of my seizure activity, especially the seizure at the choir festival just days earlier,

though I did tell him. The only thing he told my father and myself was how he couldn't raise the

Oxcarbazepine because of the dosage. He only told us how my body would adjust, and how a

breakthrough seizure was going to occur once in a while. We trusted Doctor Michaels; I trusted

Doctor Michaels.

. . . . .

I received an email that told me that I would be going to Sacramento from March 20-22,

2014 for the All-State Honor Choir. The All-State Honor Choir is where they choose the "top" students from the Southern, Central, and Northern regional choirs to perform in one choir. I would again be in the Men's Choir, but I was happy. So, my mother, sisters, and me took a giant road trip to Northern California so I could perform. Breezy also went, where she would sing in the Mixed Choir this time. The All-State Honor Choir was the highlight of our spring break. Both of our families spent the whole time together.

When we got back to school the following week, Miss Evans told everyone in all of the choirs how the two of us went to the All-State Honor Choir. Breezy and I had become irritated, so we had left the choir room without her noticing, and we just talked outside for a while. But it had started again. I felt that funny feeling. I froze and Breezy knew what was happening. She helped me sit down so we could wait it out. It eventually ended, and Miss Evans came out and asked us why we were outside.

"Uh, Jimmy just had a seizure." Breezy told her

"You two need to come back inside. He can sit down in here. I'll get him water sweetheart."

Breezy and I walked back inside the choir room and rejoined the rest of the class, their eyes fixed on both of us. I sat the rest of rehearsal. I felt out of place sitting but I did anyway. Miss Evans came back into the room with a bottle of water and handed it to me, then went to the piano to warm up the choir.

HOPE WITHIN ME

During March that year, my hopes were low. With multiple seizures every month I felt defeated. I wanted it to stop. But I knew I needed to be optimistic. I knew if there would be moving forward, I needed to put faith somewhere. Whether it was Doctor Michaels, God, somewhere. It wasn't easy for me to do that year.

What came in the mail that month snowballed into something that gave me a spark of hope again. On March 5, 2014, I had received my first letter from the small Liberal Arts College. I had been granted acceptance. I still needed to wait and hear about the audition from the School of Music though, that was what really mattered to me.

TUESDAY, MARCH 11, 2014

It wasn't long after I received the first admission letter from the Liberal Arts College before I received the news about how my audition had gone. It took approximately one week after I received my first letter before I received the second letter, this time from the School of Music. I was terrified to open it, as I has been accepted to the Liberal Arts College, but still needed to be accepted to the School of Music itself in order to pursue the degree I wanted.

I stood in the kitchen of our house; both of my parents waited for the answer. My mother, who had taken me to voice and theory lessons for a whole year wanted to know the results. I knew they wouldn't have been disappointed either way. But for myself, I didn't want the disappointment, but I knew I needed to look at it eventually. So, I opened the letter. It read:

JAMES VALENCIA

Dear James,

Congratulations! On behalf of the Faculty of the School of Music, I am writing to notify

you that you have been accepted to the School of Music to pursue the Bachelor of Music

degree. You have been accepted for applied study on Voice.

The audition committee has also recommended you for a Music Scholarship. That

recommendation has been made to the Director of Financial Aid for consideration with

any other awards, which you may be eligible, and for inclusion in your financial aid.

Music Scholarships are renewed annually up to a maximum of four years subject to

university guidelines, which include maintaining a minimum cumulative grade point

average of 3.0 (on a 4.0 scale), taking private lessons and participation in a large

ensemble (Band, Orchestra, or Choir).

We hope you find that joining us is a rewarding, musical, and academic experience.

Sincerely,

Director of Music Admissions

School of Music

After I read the letter, I couldn't believe it. I had actually been accepted to the Liberal Arts

College and School of Music. I was excited and wanted to go there! I told Miss Evans when I

saw her. She hugged me and congratulated me. She told everyone in every choir, and how proud

64

she was of me. At that moment, it felt like everything had disappeared, like my health didn't

even exist. Like if I were to go to that school, I could start over, a new page, clean.

. . . . .

From March through May of 2014, my parents and I spent a lot of time talking about how

we could afford that school and how I could get there since I didn't drive. My parents agreed to

let me go to the small Liberal Arts College, because they knew my passion was music and that I

had worked hard all year to get accepted there. We made the final decision in May; I would go

and pursue my Bachelor of Music degree at the Liberal Arts College.

With high school Graduation in June, it felt surreal to be done with my four years at the

high school. My true first public school. Graduation came and went. Many good-byes, tears, and

a few graduation parties. Nothing excited me more than to start college.

INSURANCE - JUNE 2014

HIGH SCHOOL WAS OVER, and I had just turned 18 years old. It was time for another appointment with Doctor Michaels. The insurance had given my parents problems all that month. My parents had come to find out, because I had just turned of legal age, the insurance was no longer covering me at the *Medical Center*. So, I was not be able to see Doctor Michaels, the specialist anymore, and I needed to see a general adult neurologist at the small medical group again. My parents had tried to fight it, but it was a battle they could not win. I was no longer a pediatric patient anymore; I was 18 years old and I needed to deal with it.

My parents and I were nervous about moving back to the small medical group, but it seemed like we had no other choice. I was now with the small medical group with a different doctor. His name was Doctor Klark, and he was older than Doctor Michaels and wasn't an

JAMES VALENCIA

Epilepsy specialist, just a general neurologist. However, he knew more than the first neurologist I had ever seen with that small medical group. He kept me on the *Oxcarbazepine* and the same dosage as Doctor Michaels since it had worked up to that point. The new neurologist was nice, but the appointments weren't as frequent as they were with Doctor Michaels. Instead of every two or three months, appointments were to be in six-month increments. My parents and I prayed that the new general neurologist was going to be able to help with my Epilepsy.

II

. . . . .

COLLEGE ORIENTATION WEEK

FRESHMAN YEAR OF COLLEGE had begun. It was Orientation Week, August 27 –

September 1, 2014, which was the week before classes had started, where all the students and

professors would get to meet each other. Nervous and excited, I walked around the campus of the

Liberal Arts College when I decided to go to the School of Music and look around the building.

It was the only time I had actually been inside since my audition back in February, as it was early

September at that point. The building was just as small as I had remembered it to be.

I heard a woman laughing from one of the front offices in the building. I stopped to sit on

a couch that was in the hallway to listen and try to make out the conversation. They were talking

about the *FYS* class, and how she was one of the instructors. There were classes required that

music students needed to take throughout their undergraduate, and *FYS* was one, along with:

JAMES VALENCIA

First Year Seminar (FYS) - Freshman Only

Class Piano

Music Theory I,II,III,IV

Ear Training I,II, III,IV

Private Lessons (Respective Instrument)

Ensemble (Band, Orchestra, or Choir)

Music History

These were just some of the general requirements for the Bachelor of Music degree. To what extent they needed to be finished depended on the emphasis of your degree.

However, after overhearing the woman talk, she had mentioned the choirs, and how she was ready to start rehearsals with the *Mixed Auditioned Singers*. *Mixed Auditioned Singers* was the premier mixed choir at the college. This intrigued me when I heard this.

She was the choral conductor of Mixed Auditioned Singers! I thought to myself.

I should introduce myself to her and make a good impression.

When I saw her walk out of the front office onto the front patio, I would go and take the chance, not knowing how foolish I might look. She was wearing a blue dress and earrings when I first met her. I went up to introduce myself.

"Good morning, I'm James. But I go by Jimmy." I said as politely as I could.

"Good morning Jimmy. It's nice to meet you. My name is Dr. Anders, I'm the Director of

74

Choral Studies here and one of the choral conductors." She replied.

I was nervous, and even more scared and I knew she could tell.

"I went to one of the local high schools not far from here and sang in choir." I told her.

"That's great! We'll see you at choir auditions then?" Dr. Anders asked.

"Yes, I can't wait!" I replied.

" Great! See you then Jimmy." She said hurriedly before she walked away.

I felt confident at that point. Classes hadn't event begun and I had met the conductor of

Mixed Auditioned Singers and the Director of Choral Studies.

CLASSES BEGIN - MONDAY, SEPTEMBER 2, 2014

The morning of actual classes had arrived. It started with me sitting in my living room, it was five thirty in the morning. I always needed to get up that early because I still didn't drive due to my Epilepsy. So, the deal I had made with my parents back in May was that I would ride my bicycle to college, and my father would pick me up in his truck in the evening after he would get off of work. I remember sitting on the living room couch drinking my coffee staring at my music theory textbook, excited and nervous. I ate a nutritious breakfast, toast, and eggs, before shoving my textbook into my backpack at six thirty and heading out the door to ride to the college. I had practiced the ride before to time it out, because there was too much traffic riding past my old high school in the morning hours, so it was perfect timing. It took me between twenty-five and thirty minutes to get there, so I would be there around seven in the morning. I liked to be early to finish last minute homework in the mornings. Riding my bicycle to school the first week was working out great. It was calming in a sense. My parents enjoyed it too because they only needed to pick me up in the evenings, so it worked out for all of us.

That first week of classes was an important week for all the choirs and vocalists. It was audition week. There were three choirs at the Liberal Arts College. There were two premier choirs, the *Mixed Auditioned Singers*, which represented the college most of the time, and the *Women's Auditioned Choir*. Then, there was *General Choir* that was non-auditioned where anyone could join. The two premier choirs usually took around twenty-four to thirty voices, and *General Choir* took almost double or more voices at times.

Having been in the top choir in high school had made me think the audition process would be easy in college, and I could make *Mixed Auditioned Singers* my freshman year. When I walked into the audition room, there were only two people in there. Dr. Anders, who I had met the week prior, and Dr. Marino, the assistant Director of Choral Studies and the choral conductor of the *Women's Auditioned Choir* and *General Choir*. I was asked to vocalize for them, and sang for tonal memory, then was given a rhythm and sight-reading. It would be at that moment I started to realize I knew nothing about sight-reading or musicianship. That year, after the audition process, I was placed in *General Choir*.

September went by, and October had finally arrived. I had started to realize that being a fulltime college music student was difficult. I was taking more classes than the average college student, as I had private lessons and choir on top of my seven normal classes.

. . . . . .

It was a normal morning in October, while riding my bicycle to the college I had felt a funny feeling. I was over halfway to the college and knew I was probably less than a mile and a half away, so I didn't want to stop. I ignored the feeling and kept riding. I started to feel myself get a freezing sensation, so I tried to pull over to the sidewalk, but it was too late. I found myself with an older couple who gave me a water bottle. They explained to me that they had seen me fall onto their fence and into their yard with my bicycle. I told them thank you for the water and for their help.

I got back onto my bicycle to finish the journey to the college, as I was determined to go to class. When I had arrived at the college, I went straight to the bathroom, and while in there I noticed my shirt had a tear on my sleeve. There was also a giant cut on my upper bicep, which I would still have the scar years later. I sat in the bathroom of the building for a few minutes and cried. I cried at how dumb I must have looked, and what my peers would think, and why it had happened to me on a school day, or at all. I realized there were only minutes before class would start, so I started to walk to my first class of the day with a torn sleeve.

My first class that day was *Ear Training I* with Dr. Anders. We were all sitting down in our seats, Dr. Anders sat at a table in front of the classroom to write on the board and speak, I sat somewhere in the middle trying to avoid being seen by anyone, though no one really talked to me much freshman year anyway. In *Ear Training I*, we would do practice and prepared sight-readings, and it was my turn to go up. I will never forget that moment in my life. All my peers staring at me as I slowly made my way up to the front of the classroom.

"Jimmy, what happened to your arm?" She asked me, looking at my ripped sleeve.

I felt embarrassed, ashamed. No one at the college knew about my Epilepsy, and I didn't want anyone to know. I wanted a clean slate. I was determined to keep it that way.

"I was attacked by a squirrel." I replied. Chuckling a little.

We had many squirrels on the campus. The comment seemed to make the rest of the class ignore her question and laugh which made me feel less embarrassed, however I was still ashamed of my health internally.

"Oh, okay." She said. Obviously, she had not believed me.

"Let's look at the sight-reading." She had me continue.

When I had finished with the sight-reading, I quickly sat down in my seat in the middle of the class to try and disappear again. The rest of class went by fast, and I was able to go to my next class. I hurried out to my next class, *Class Piano*. Though, on the walk to my next class, I noticed my right toe was hurting. I was wearing sandals that day, so when I looked down, I had noticed it bleeding with the whole big toenail hanging off. No one had noticed, and I hadn't either. I had scraped it when I fell. So, I cleaned it in a bathroom, then went to *Class Piano* and played the best I could. Before long it started to hurt more. I eventually told my Piano instructor I had scraped my toenail "somehow" and needed to leave class. She had excused me from the rest of class that day. When I left the class, I immediately called my father and told him, over the phone, what had happened that morning. He came to pick me up and we both went to urgent care to get my toe taken care of. The whole toenail was wrapped up and I was given a boot as a support for my toe. I wore that boot for a week.

After the incident on my bicycle, I was determined to keep my Epilepsy and seizures a secret from my professors and peers at the college. I didn't know how they would react or what they would think of me if they knew. I felt lonely for many months my freshman year, going to all my classes, *Music Theory I, Ear Training I, FYS, Class Piano, Voice Lessons, Choir,* only praying I would never have a seizure in front of anyone. Never making friends. I would take my lunch up to a practice room where I would lock myself in there to eat and wait for my next class, and once classes were over for the day, I would go straight home. Never socializing, scared to let someone get close.

WEDNESDAY, DECEMBER 3, 2014

As the first semester came to an end, the School of Music was preparing for its annual Christmas

performance it gave the first week of every December. Most of the music majors and students in

the choirs and orchestra spent the week prior to the performance rehearsing almost every night.

All three choirs, the orchestra, the two choral conductors, and a guest conductor were performing

that year. We had found out a few weeks earlier, the guest conductor that year would be the

Chancellor of the Liberal Arts College. He was going to be conducting *Hallelujah Chorus* from

Handel's Messiah. The choirs were to process into the building while singing it. So, as the choirs

were rehearsing and practiced the processing at one of the rehearsal nights, the Chancellor

happened to be standing in front of me and conducting while I sang and processed in towards the

stage. However, I felt that funny feeling. Without any time to react, I was half sitting and laying on top of the Chancellor. I fell and had a seizure on the Chancellor of the college. I couldn't remember who, but Dr. Anders or Dr. Marino continued conducting *Hallelujah Chorus* for the Chancellor so the rehearsal could continue, and they could divert the attention away.

I sat in the audience seats the rest of rehearsal, never making it to the actual stage from the procession that rehearsal night. Someone I knew from high school, involved in instrumental music, informed Dr. Anders, and the Chancellor it was a seizure I had. In the middle of rehearsal, when everyone was given a break to rest, the Chancellor and Dr. Anders came over to me. I was scared, not knowing what to expect.

"How are you feeling Jimmy? Or do you prefer James?" the Chancellor asked me.

"You can call me Jimmy, and I feel good, just tired." I replied.

"So, you just had a seizure? That's what a young fellow in one of the ensembles that knows you told us." He continued to ask me.

"Yes, I did. I'm sorry that I fell on you." I told him.

"Don't be sorry, luckily there were people around to help." He said.

I wanted to cry, just disappear, or to go home and lay in my bed. I had felt bad I had fallen on the Chancellor, and in front of everyone in the rehearsal. What I had tried to keep a secret, I felt like everyone would soon know.

"Is it caused by anything in particular?" He asked.

"I think stress and sleep sometimes, but I'm not certain."

HOPE WITHIN ME

"Well, I'll tell you what, and this will always be in place for you if you need it during this time of the year. With finals week approaching and this stressful time of the year, if you need more time on anything such as homework assignments, papers, projects, or finals, let me know. Or have Dr. Anders let me know and I'll email your professors directly and tell them to give you more time."

The Chancellor said this with a sincere face to me and Dr. Anders who stood there as well. All I could do in that moment was stare at him and nod.

"You hear that Jimmy, just let either the Chancellor know, or you let me know and I'll email the Chancellor for you." Dr. Anders agreeing to what the Chancellor had just told me.

Rehearsal would soon start with Dr. Marino again. I sat out the rest of that rehearsal making marks in my vocal score, trying not to feel self-conscious knowing other students would notice I was sitting out in the audience seats. But finally, after many rehearsal nights that year, the Christmas performances came the following week. It had turned out great. It was one of the most spectacular performances I had been a part of, and knowing it happened every year, I would be able to try it again the following year without any incidents. I was still nervous and scared that everyone knew of my health condition though.

However, finals week was stressful but a success, and I was able to get through it without using the Chancellor's offer and receive decent grades, especially for the first semester of college. My first semester in college and as a music major went good other than the seizure

85

that exposed my health condition to a few people, but I was hopeful nobody would remember after Christmas break and it would eventually fade in everyone's memory.

. . . . .

It had been about six months since my last visit with Doctor Klark, my new general neurologist, and I now had an appointment. Visits with him were different compared to the specialist, and they were also shorter. I went in, and he asked if I had any episodes (seizures). I listed all of the seizures I had during the fall and I described them to him, gave him the dates and that was it. He hadn't said much or given me any feedback. Being in the adult neurology was different, as I would go into my appointments alone. This appointment lasted only twenty or twenty-five minutes before it ended, and we said our good-byes.

THE TALK - SPRING 2015

JANUARY 2015 of my freshman year of college, and it was a new semester. I felt refreshed from the three-week Christmas break I just had. I was ready to take on a brand-new semester. The last semester of my first year of college, hoping those few people who knew of my Epilepsy had forgotten over their Christmas break so I could continue to hide it and try to appear to live a "normal" life to the people at the Liberal Arts College.

It was time for me to go to my *Ear Training II* class, as most freshman completed level I during the first semester. We went about the same material and routine only harder. This class was also be taught by Dr. Anders, she taught levels I and II. The class was being dismissed as the scheduled time was over, and most students needed to go to their next class or wanted to go about their day. That's when she walked over to me, waited for students to leave and asked if there was a time her and Dr. Marino could talk to me. Dr. Anders assured me I wasn't in trouble, as I must've looked terrified. The three of us scheduled to meet later that afternoon in the front office to talk privately.

It had seemed as if no one had forgotten about December, especially the two people I wanted. Before I met with them, all I could think about was how they viewed me. I could only imagine what we were going to discuss. Before I went to the office, I sat on the couch outside in the hallway. It was the same couch I sat on during orientation week. Finally, I saw Dr. Anders and Dr. Marino walk into the building together. I stood up and smiled, a half fake smile to try and hold back the disappointment in my heart.

"Hi Jimmy, how are you doing?" Dr. Marino asked, with a smile.

He always had the brightest smiles.

Dr. Anders was trying to unlock the front office door.

"I'm good Dr. Marino. How about you?" I replied.

Dr. Anders finally opened the door to the front office.

"I'm great. Thanks." Dr. Marino said before he walked into the office.

"Hello Jimmy, come on inside."

Dr. Anders said, letting me into the office before she shut the door behind her.

I had only been in the front office a few times. There were two long, black leather couches, mailboxes belonging to professors, and the Director of Music Admissions desk. The two leather couches were parallel and faced each other. Dr. Anders and Dr. Marino both sat on

one that was against the wall and I sat on the opposite couch, so we all faced each other.

I was nervous, knowing why we were there and what the discussion was about. I tried my

best not to make eye contact with either of them, but only with the abstract piece of artwork that

hung on the wall above their couch. Then, I heard Dr. Marino start to speak:

"So, Jimmy, we wanted to meet with you because in December you had an incident at the

Christmas performance rehearsal." He continued.

"We aren't *legally* allowed to ask you anything about your health, but wanted to know if

there's anything Dr. Anders or myself can do if it were to happen again?"

"Uh, I just need to sit down. Maybe get a drink of water. I can usually go right back to

what I was doing before. I don't remember anything during my seizure though." I told them.

"Did you get that Dr. Anders, help him sit down and water." He repeated to her.

"Do any of your peers know about this or that you have seizures?" Dr. Anders asked me.

"No." I replied, as I tried not to make eye contact with either of them.

"Do you mind if we ask you why?" Dr. Marino asked.

"I just didn't want anyone to know about it."

"Are you embarrassed by it?" Dr. Anders asked me.

Part of me wanted to be honest and say "yes" but I had stayed quiet for a while, which I

knew gave a definite answer to both of them, before I gave a plain answer.

"I don't know. I just didn't want anyone here knowing." I told them.

"Having a health condition isn't something to be embarrassed or ashamed of. There are students and faculty members here at the School of Music who have health conditions. *I* have one, and you wouldn't even know it." Dr. Anders told me.

"You see Jimmy, we all want to be here for you, and we all have our issues. The School of Music is a good place for that, as you can see." Dr. Marino said.

All three of us laughed a little.

"Let us know how we can help you. You don't need to hide your seizures or Epilepsy if you don't want to." Dr. Anders told me.

"Plus aren't you Jimmy's academic advisor Dr. Marino?"

"Yes, I am. So, let me know if you ever need anything, okay Jimmy? Just email me or Dr. Anders." Dr. Marino said with a smile.

When the meeting was over, and we were out of the tiny office, it felt weird to have talked about my Epilepsy with them. People at the college actually knew something about my health, the baggage that was a part of my life. I had tried so hard to keep it a secret, locked up. I was ashamed of it, like it was a dirty part of me, but I knew the two of them would support me. *Maybe I could open up more, even to my peers. Not about my Epilepsy quite yet, but in friendship and letting them into my life.* I thought to myself.

During that spring of freshman year, most of the guys in my freshman class were rushing a fraternity. It was a small music fraternity. I started going to all of the rush events in hopes of getting to know the guys in my freshmen class and the older guys better. I was slowly getting to know people and becoming a happier person. Most events were ultimate frisbee, capture the flag, touch football, and game nights. After many rush events, the active members of the fraternity finally chose who would go through the fraternity's process, and I was not invited to continue. I soon found out there was drama in college just like in high school. Someone from the fraternity pulled me aside and informed me I wasn't invited because they heard from another vocalist that I was arrogant and had said I was "better than another singer".

I had felt bad because that active member was nice, and the only one who invited me to all of the rush events. He wasn't even supposed to tell me why I didn't make the cut either. After that active member had informed me why I didn't make it, I told him it was false, and he could tell all of the active members it was too. I had also told him that if they chose members based on false sources than I didn't want to be a part of their fraternity. I continued to be invited to their fraternity events throughout the year anyway but ignored their invitations.

My health was no longer a secret. Two professors now knew about my Epilepsy, and I knew a few of my peers did as well. I was worried about judgement, but I needed to see how safe it truly was at the School of Music throughout my undergraduate years. It was obvious that Dr. Anders and Dr. Marino were there to offer a support to me. So, maybe if I opened myself up and let my peers and other professors into my life more during my sophomore year, I would be able to find a safe haven.

The semester and year came to its end, and instrumental and voice juries, which were performances for a panel of faculty members to see progress, had finished. I was pleased with the overall progress of my first year of music school and college.

. . . . .

It was that time again, the time where I had to meet with Doctor Klark. He was genuinely a nice person, he just didn't seem, to me, to help as much as I wanted or needed. When I met him in the spring, it was the same as the last time we had met, more taking notes, talking about how I had been feeling, and if I had any episodes or seizures. Although I was having seizures every so often, he still wouldn't do anything, he just told me, "it sounds like you have it under control". *Under control?*, was what I thought, *there was nothing under control*. But I tried to trust him as it was barely my first year with him as my neurologist. Again, we shook hands, and I left the room, unhappy of course.

CALL-BACKS - SEPTEMBER 2015 – JANUARY 2016

Fall of 2015, SOPHOMORE YEAR was here. I still only knew a few people in my actual class, so I had looked forward to going back to the School of Music to try and make friends in the upcoming academic year. It was the first week of September, the week before classes actually began. However, choir auditions were being held a week early because *Mixed Auditioned Singers* were going to Portland Oregon for a competition in early November. Dr. Anders had hard music for them to learn and memorize by mid-October and needed to book their plane tickets that week. Dr. Anders and Dr. Marino had decided to audition differently that year. They auditioned everyone for choir as usual, and then narrowed it down to a call-back system. I was shocked, I had been placed on the call-back list. The call-backs were going to be held the next day in the performance hall, where I had originally auditioned for the School of Music.

I stared at the call-back list in shock when a member of the previous year's tenor section in *Mixed Auditioned Singers* saw me and started to talk to me.

"I've heard you sing before and you have a great tone quality. You'll definitely get into *Mixed Auditioned Singers* this year." He told me before he glanced back at the list.

"You think? I'm not a strong sight-reader though."

"You'll definitely get in. You see this guy?" He pointed to another tenor. "He told Dr. Anders and all of *Mixed Auditioned Singers* he couldn't go to a performance because he was "sick", then we all found out he wasn't sick, he went to a concert instead." He told me.

I was shocked. Someone had lied to Dr. Anders and the choir. Who would do that?

"You'll get in, don't worry about it." He patted me on the back before walking away.

He had said nice compliments, but after talking with the tenor, I tried not to give my hopes up before call-back day. When it came time for call-backs the next day, everyone was in the performance hall. I was relieved there was no sight-reading involved. Dr. Anders and Dr. Marino only focused on blending and had groups of quartets in front of them. They listened closely. I was shocked because I was up there almost the entire time, like they had purposely put students next to me. When call-backs had finally ended, we waited as the two choral conductors made the final list. They posted it quickly to the wall by the front office. After I scanned the tenor section multiple times, I didn't find my name. I looked at the *General Choir* list and found my name there. I was disappointed and wanted to cry. I went to the patio and sat

94

on a bench. The tenor who had spoken to me the day before found me outside. He came up to me, gave me a side hug and apologized. He told me how much I deserved to be there instead of the other tenor. Although I just wanted to go home and not speak about it, I told him it was fine. I went home later that afternoon, went up to my bedroom and cried. I cried for over thirty minutes before I realized I could trust Dr. Anders and Dr. Marino. They knew my voice and had seen me grow throughout my freshman year. They both knew my musicianship and knew what I could and couldn't sing.

Throughout September and October, I came to realize that being in *General Choir* was more beneficial than being in *Mixed Auditioned Singers*. I saw how even the more advanced singers struggled with music and memorization; I couldn't have possibly dealt with that. I also noticed how I was opening up to people in my own class. I had started making friends. I started staying at school later, eating lunch with other students, and practicing homework assignments for music classes. It became fun being a music student.

Once again, it was time for the annual Christmas performances at the Liberal Arts College, hosted by the School of Music. The end of November and beginning of December was always busy for music majors and faculty. But as stressful as it always was, the facility on the campus we used for the performance was always beautiful. It was filled with evergreen branches that smelled like Christmas.

After the previous year's incident with the Chancellor, I was scared it would happen again. However, I was able to get through the whole week of rehearsals without a single incident or seizure. It was the last night of the Christmas performance, and most of us music majors were tired of singing or playing instruments but glad it was the last performance. Intermission had just ended, and it was the second half of the performance. Dr. Marino was about to conduct and he had gestured for the choirs to stand, so we all stood, and the orchestra started to play. We took a deep breath, and we started to sing.

As we sang in beautiful harmony, there it was, that funny feeling, that sensation. Although there were benches for the whole choir to sit, I stayed standing trying to ignore it. I didn't want attention brought in my direction. I looked to my right, and Dr. Anders was sitting on stage right against the wall in a chair, where the conductors sat when they weren't conducting. She saw me, so without hesitation or anyone noticing, she started to crawl on her hands and knees through the choirs and benches over to me and sat with me to make sure I was okay. As soon as my seizure was over, she asked if I was okay to keep singing. I told her I could, that I *wanted* to keep singing. She then discretely made her way back to stage right through backstage from the stage left door while everyone clapped, and the orchestra stood to bow. When I arrived home that night, I laid in bed and just stared at the ceiling. I couldn't believe it. It was the first time I had ever had a seizure during a performance. I was embarrassed, my professor had crawled on her hands and knees to come help me.

It was soon finals week again. As finals week approached, a tenor, the same tenor who had said I would make *Mixed Auditioned Singers*, asked a group of guys if we wanted to create a Men's Choir for the college. Excitedly, I signed up. All the guys brought the list to both the choral conductors in December, and Dr. Anders decided she would be the choral conductor. We started the first ever Men's Choir for the college. Rehearsals started in January; they were interesting. Most of the guys in the choir were instrumentalists, so some of the music wasn't too hard, but the music chosen was fun and level appropriate.

In the middle of January 2016, I was given multiple invitations to rush for the music fraternity again. I had kept denying them, still upset at the accusations from the previous year, but eventually I had decided to forgive them and give them a chance to see what they were about. I had figured that since I was a music major and knew a majority of the members better compared to the previous year, it was worth trying.

After many rush events that month, I had started to wonder if I was even going to be considered for the fraternity. On a Friday, while I walked to class, an active member walked up to me, handed me a tiny piece of white paper folded up into fours, then walked away. It read:

Dear James Valencia,

You are invited to the formal rush for the music fraternity Sunday, January 25th, 2016 at 9:30pm. Please present yourself in formal attire at our fraternity's house.

Sincerely,

The brothers of the music fraternity

I was excited when I had received the invitation. They were selective on who they wanted for this event, and I made it. Before I went to the event, I lied to my parents and told them I needed to practice at the college. So, my father dropped me off, with a suit, at five o'clock in the evening and I waited until it was time for the event. I'm not sure why my parents hadn't noticed the suit with me. But I went that Sunday night to the formal event. After the event had finished, a friend I had met there, who was also rushing, was nice enough to drive me home. When I arrived home, I fell asleep not knowing what to think. I waited, not knowing if I would receive a bid for the actual fraternity process.

It wasn't until sometime during the following week that I received a bid from the fraternity. Those of us who received these bids and were interested in continuing were taken to a secret location. My new fraternity class stood there in a row and waited to receive our Big Brothers. The President of the fraternity talked to us about secret information before he told us to turn around to see our new Big Brothers. Our Big Brother's responsibility was to help guide us through the fraternity process and to be there for us when we needed it.

I turned around, and there was no one there. I looked down the line at everyone else in my new fraternity class, and they all had their Big Brothers. I stood there alone.

This can't be right. Maybe because I distanced myself from so many people last year nobody wanted to be my Big Brother. I thought to myself.

I kept looking, not straying from the row we were to stay in. Then, suddenly I felt someone tap me on my shoulder. I slowly turned around, and it was the President of the fraternity. I was scared for a second before he started to speak.

"Hey Little!" He said vibrantly before he gave me a giant hug.

"Sorry I'm late, as you could see, I was speaking." He said.

"That's okay, I was just confused." I muttered out, trying not to sound nervous.

Little? The President was my Big Brother? I couldn't believe it; my Big Brother was the President of the fraternity. I hadn't been forgotten after all.

Soon, all of us were headed to get food to bring back to the fraternity house, with the Big Brothers buying for their Littles. It amazed me at how kind everyone in the fraternity was. There I was, an outcast the previous year. I had distanced myself, and now they were buying me food.

ALLERGIC REACTION - FEBRUARY 2016

It was a normal *Music History* class in February at eight in the morning. Everyone was sitting in

their seats waiting for Dr. Bailey, the musicologist, to arrive and start the lecture for the day.

Most mornings, students brought their breakfast or coffee into the classroom and would eat and

drink it during the lecture, and Dr. Bailey would be fine with it. After that day, which no one

could have foreseen, no one felt comfortable doing so. We were probably ten minutes into the

lecture. I was sitting somewhere in the middle of the classroom, as I liked to see the board

because Dr. Bailey used it a lot. I suddenly realized she had stopped the lecture and was looking

my way. I had thought she was thinking I was having a seizure. I instinctively started to shake

my head and tried to mouth the words *I'm fine* to her. I started to look around the classroom. I

had noticed a few other of my peers looking my way as well, but I couldn't tell if they were looking at me or something else. I then noticed what they were looking at. They weren't looking at me, they were looking at our friend Tina. Only a few people in the room had noticed, she was having an allergic reaction. Tina was allergic to something someone had brought into the room, and she was having an anaphylactic reaction. Dr. Bailey and a few peers noticed right away. We cleared the desks and helped Tina onto the floor and used one of two Epinephrine injectors she always carried two in her back pocket. However, the first wasn't enough, but we didn't want to inject the second as it could cause cardiac arrest. A student ran to the classroom next door, where Dr. Marino was teaching beginning conducting at the time to inform him what was happening. He came running over and we immediately called the paramedics. Tina was taken to the hospital.

Tina came out of the hospital later that night with Dr. Anders, who had been kind enough to go visit and pick her up. I sat and talked with Tina about everything the following day on the patio. She told me how embarrassed she felt because she stopped class. When she told me that, it resonated with me.

"I feel like that too with my seizures. Like with my seizure during the Christmas performance. It was embarrassing, Dr. Anders crawling to me." I told her.

"But you can't control that. That's not your fault." Tina replied.

"Neither is your allergy though. If someone brings in a certain food without you knowing, that's not your fault either."

"It just sucked having everyone stare at me, and then having the class stopped."

"I feel the same way at times. I know it brings attention to me. Plus, we were more concerned about your safety, not what we were learning about" I told her.

"I never thought about that. We think about that with your seizures too. I guess we both think alike when it comes to our health." Tina said with a small smile.

"I never knew you thought the same way either. I hope you're feeling better Tina."

We both stood up and hugged each other and went on with our day. It was the first time I had a heart to heart with Tina, and with another peer about my health and Epilepsy in general. Someone who actually felt the same way that I did.

After the next *Music History* class, I had decided it would be important to sit down and talk with Dr. Bailey. So, the two of us sat on the front patio of the School of Music at the college to talk.

"Good morning Dr. Bailey" I started by saying.

"Good morning Jimmy. What's on your mind?" She asked, sipping her cup of coffee.

"I wanted to talk to you about my seizures. As you probably already know, I have Epilepsy, a type of seizure disorder."

She just nodded and smiled politely.

"I talked to Tina, and we had a heart to heart about our health. And it's hard sometimes, because it can feel like I can be a burden on everyone here at the school when I have a seizure, and I don't try to be." My eyes started to water at that point, so I looked down.

I felt Dr. Bailey get closer to me, and then felt her hand on my back.

"Jimmy, your seizures are not your fault. And you are not a burden to me or anyone in the School of Music." She said.

"I just feel like I'm in the way sometimes, annoying people when I have a seizure."

"Your health is not your fault, just like Tina's health, or what happened in class with her, wasn't her fault. You can't control when you have a seizure. You have all of these people, like Dr. Anders, Dr. Marino, Tina, and me who want to be there for you, just let us know how we can help you, okay?"

She said it with a smile, as tears ran down my face. She gave me a half hug before we both stood up so she could go inside and teach her second *Music History* class of that day.

"You have a good day Jimmy."

"Thank you Dr. Bailey. You too." I said, trying to hold back the rest of my tears.

I was amazed I had that heart to heart with Dr. Bailey. So, I decided since I had no classes for the rest of that morning, I would go to the library's computer center to type up instructions for my School of Music professors in case I were to have a seizure in their class. It would take a good amount of time to complete the instructions for my professors, but when it was complete, I wanted it to be thorough. It would explain what Epilepsy was, what my specific type of seizure looked like, what happens before my seizures, what happens after my seizures, and what the faculty members should do during the seizures.

HOPE WITHIN ME

The 2016 letter and instructions given to School of Music faculty. It read:

Dear faculty,

My name is Jimmy Valencia. I am writing to inform you of my Epileptic (seizure) condition. The Type I have is referred to as Partial Complex seizures. Below is information on what a seizure is, as well as instructions on what to do if one should occur. Thank you for taking the time to read this and your willingness to accommodate my medical condition throughout my time here, ensuring my academic success.

What is Epilepsy?

Epilepsy is a neurological disorder, and it starts and occurs in the brain. During a Seizure, there are bursts of electrical activity in the brain, sort of like an electrical storm.

What do my seizures look like?

During the seizure, I will not remember what occurs throughout the entirety of the event. I may move, see, or do normal things. It will appear that I am looking out into space, or that I am under the influence of some sort. I may also drool as well.

What happens before my seizures?

There are no visual signs for anyone else before a seizure takes place. For myself though, I have an "aura", or warning, before a seizure. An aura is a change in feeling, sensation, thought, or behavior. They will often happen before the main part of the seizure.

What happens after a seizure?

After a seizure, I will usually be able to go back to the task I was doing before. I will most likely be sleepy or tired since the seizure causes exhaustion.

Instruction during the seizure

1. *Stay calm*

2. *DO NOT call an ambulance (the only reason to call for an ambulance is if I am shaking violently or it lasts longer than 5 minutes)*

3. *DO NOT put anything in my mouth, that is more of a choking hazard*

4. *Make sure I am sitting down somewhere*

5. *Stay with me until the seizure is over*

6. *Keep track of how long it lasts*

When the letter and instructions were finished, I made multiple copies. One copy of the letter and instructions were put into every School of Music professor's mailbox in the front office.

CHOIR SOLO - MARCH 2016

It was the middle of March, and the Men's Choir had still only given one performance, which was at the choral concert earlier in the semester. We were learning a fun piece, *Manly Men* by Kurt Knecht, and I was to have a solo. It was being conducted by one of the Master's of Music Conducting students, so Dr. Anders wanted it to be performed. It would also give the ensemble exposure, so we were scheduled to perform it for a group of our music peers on a Wednesday. I was excited, as I had been practicing for months at that point and would get to sing up to a high "C" on my solo.

The time of the performance had arrived. Our peers sat in the audience, waiting for the performance, as we stood behind a grey curtain on stage right, anticipating what we would sound like to them. We started to walk onto the stage, into two semi-circles, each behind each other facing the audience. The conductor walked out a few seconds later, gestured for us to bow,

then walked in front of us and raised her hands. She took a deep breath with us, and we began to

sing. She looked at me, gave a slight nod of her head, that was the cue for me to walk up and

sing the solo. Not nervous at all, I sang through it with ease, singing through the high "C". As

my solo ended, I felt it again. There it was, the funny feeling and sensation. The difference was it

happened fast. I had actually tried to leave the stage, since I was already at the edge, and the

stage was not raised, but level with the ground and seats, but I couldn't make it. There was

another student who saw me and immediately helped me sit down. When the seizure was over, I

had realized I was sitting with a cup of water in my hand and everyone was clapping for the

Men's Choir as I sat in the back of the audience. Embarrassed, I left the room during the

clapping. This had been the second time during the year I had a seizure during a performance. I

didn't know what student had helped me, I sat on the couch out by the front office when I heard

a student's voice ask me a question.

"Are you feeling better" She asked.

"Yeah, I'm feeling better, just embarrassed, that's all." I said.

It was another Master's of Music student. She had seen me start to wonder off stage during the

performance. That must have been when I had tried to sit down, having the aura, but didn't have

time to sit. She had helped guide me to a seat in the back and got me water.

"Don't be embarrassed. I saw you and wanted to make sure you were okay." She told me.

In that moment I wanted to cry. I was barely able to get through a solo before having a seizure in front of all of my peers. They all knew what my Epilepsy and seizures now looked like.

"Thank you. I have Epilepsy, so I was having a seizure." I continued to tell her.

Going about the rest of the day, I had wanted to forget about the performance and the seizure, as it had brought another wave of guilt and shame over me.

SOFTBALLFEILD - WEDNESDAY, MARCH 10, 2016

All I could think about was the fraternity and the events, as most of the week was filled with their requirements. I could honestly say that without the members in my new fraternity class, going through the process would have been harder than it *actually* was.

Throughout the spring semester of 2016, I lied to my parents about why I stayed late at the college. I ended up telling them I was "practicing" for classes, which would be accurate at times, or that I needed to use the computer center. They never questioned it, as I wouldn't let them know I was rushing a fraternity that year. Since I was making friends sophomore year, I was getting rides at night after our fraternity events. I was getting close to people in my fraternity class, like Kris, who was a year younger than me and a music minor. There was Theo, who was also younger than me and played trumpet and was a music education major. They would both give me rides home after events. I also made a friend named Jeff that year, he was a music composition major, who wasn't going through Process like Kris, Theo, or myself, but also offered to give me a ride home if I ever needed it. It had felt good going through process that spring. I had been making friends and getting close to people.

It was a busy Wednesday night, where the new fraternity class had an event. A last-minute task needed to be done for me, so I headed to the fraternity house. I had been waiting until the last minute to get a task completed compared to the rest of my fraternity class. To get to the fraternity house, you needed to pass the baseball and softball fields. It had been dark at that time and it was eight or eight thirty at night, but I needed the task completed. Walking with my music binder in my hands, I was alone on my way. I was crossing the softball field, as I was trying to make it in a faster time. I started to feel funny. That was all I had remembered before I found myself on the ground in the middle of the grass of the softball field, with my binder and papers spread out on the ground twenty feet away. I stood up, staring, and looking around. It was a dark part of the campus where no one went at night, so no one had seen me. I went to pick up the binder and papers, only to debate on going to the fraternity house. I ended up sitting on the softball field bleachers and cried at my shame. I had known some of the active members knew of my Epilepsy, but to what extent I hadn't known. I sat and cried, I knew no one could hear. Before long, I texted my Big Brother and told him I was "sick" and wasn't able to make it to the house or to the event that night. Since he was the President, he had excused me.

HOPE WITHIN ME

The next event night came. I had been scared at what I had missed at the previous event. And even more scared at what everyone would say to me. No one had known I had a seizure.

"Jimmy, we hope you're feeling better." the Fraternity Education Officer said.

"I am." I replied. Although I still felt the shame of my health on my back.

That night, the event went on. They finished the night by asking how everyone was doing. I had sat three seats away from the Fraternity Education Officer and my Big Brother.

"How are you doing with Process Jimmy?"

I had stared at the ground for a while before answering. My eyes started to water.

"I'm doing okay. The events are going fine." My throat tightened.

"I wasn't sick at the last event. I was scared to go. I had tried to go to the fraternity house the other day, and on my way," I hesitated,

"I had a seizure and found myself on the ground with my books spread out on the ground. I tried to walk to the house door but was too ashamed. I didn't want to be a burden on you guys, so I went home instead. So, I texted my Big Brother, and stayed home at the last event."

While I said this, tears streamed down my face, and I was barely able to speak the words, but instead forced them out. It was silent for a minute. I had felt like the mood of the room had changed. We moved to the next two guys in my class before we had finally reached the Fraternity Education Officer.

"Thank you everyone. I just want to let you know," he paused and looked at me.

"None of you are a burden on us. We consider you brothers. Jimmy, if you would have knocked on the fraternity house door that night, we would have welcomed you in with open arms. We love you brother. You are not a burden." He said as he came to hug me.

I soon felt another embrace from behind me.

"I love you Little. You are not a burden." It was my Big Brother

Soon, all of the active members surrounded me, along with my own fraternity class, all of them hugged me and said the same thing, "We love you Jimmy, *You Are Not A Burden*."

Tears ran down my face, along with other members, who also cried. My heart felt overjoyed with the love and compassion that these men brought to me. After the event had ended, Kris was kind enough to take me home that night.

. . . . . .

As my fraternity class poured out most of our time and soul into fraternity events most of that semester, it was soon April, Initiation month. We soon became full active members of an organization that had given us so much. That had taught us, taught *me*, how to genuinely love each other and those around us. On Thursday April 21, 2016 we finally became full active members of the fraternity. It wasn't until days later I let my parents know what I had been doing throughout the semester and year with the fraternity.

HOPE WITHIN ME

. . . . . .

Sophomore year of college came to its' end. It was an emotional year, but successful in many ways. Before it ended, the announcement of the opera for the following year was emailed out by Professor Mark, Director of Opera. Going into the third year of academics at the college, I was eager to know if I could help or be a part of the production (i.e. help with staging, makeup, lighting). I received an email from Professor Mark who asked if I was interested in a lead role. Hesitant at first, and also surprised as the opera would be in French and almost two hours long, I took the opportunity. I had ten months to learn music, in French, along with other vocal music students and Professor Mark. I was excited and eager at how sophomore year had ended despite its ups and downs.

. . . . . .

I'd had four appointments at that point with Doctor Klark, and he hadn't done anything to help reduce my seizure activity. I had even met with him back in January 2016 and it had been the same as the spring of 2015 where he said, "you have it under control". But this appointment he was finally going to make a change. After listing off the seizures I had so far: the Christmas performance, the men's choir performance, and softball field where I had lost consciousness and

JAMES VALENCIA

fell, as well as all of the small ones I had throughout the year, he made the decision to change my

medication. He changed the *Oxcarbazepine* dosage. I had been taking two 600mg tablets/2x

daily but was to start taking two and a half 600mg tablets/2x daily. He wanted to see how my

body and brain would react to it. We shook hands and I was on my way out once again, except

happier because I had felt like he actually did something for the first time in two years.

SEPTEMBER 2016

It was the first week of JUNIOR YEAR OF COLLEGE. This meant that audition week was upon everyone at school, the vocalists, and instrumentalists. I was not looking forward to it as I had not been placed in the upper ensembles the previous two years and had started to doubt my ability as a musician. However, I went through the process like the past years, received a "call-back" again. At the end of this "call-back", everyone there at the time was told the list would be posted the following day. I went to look at the list, not expecting to be on it, but to my surprise, I had made it. Under the Tenor section of *Mixed Auditioned Singers*, I saw my name, Jimmy Valencia. I had felt a rush of joy go through me. The following week, I started rehearsals with the choir I had wanted to be in since I had arrived at the School of Music and the Liberal Arts College.

117

JAMES VALENCIA

Junior year would be a busy year for me and a lot of friends I had made. The previous year, I had taken an introductory music conducting course in the fall of 2015, my sophomore year, before taking an advanced choral conducting course in the spring of 2016. Having been a choral music education major, myself and three of my peers were offered to be choral conductors for the children's choir held at the college. It would be overseen and run by Dr. Anders and Dr. Marino who would help with choral conducting techniques and skills for us choral education majors. They would also give us educational advice for keeping the children engaged during the rehearsal.

It felt good for the first month and a half, until one day I had started to lose my concentration in front of the children during rehearsals. There came a point after one rehearsal where I had finished conducting and walked out of the room to get air.

"Dr. Marino, can you follow him, he might be having a seizure."

Dr. Anders asked him. "Yeah" He followed.

I had felt embarrassed. I heard Dr. Marino's footsteps coming towards me. I sat outside.

"Jimmy, are you okay?" He sat down next to me. I tried not to look at him. My eyes watered up.

"I don't know if I can do this. I'm not improving, and I feel like the children aren't learning the music as fast as they should be. How am I supposed to educate them?" I told him.

"My first year of teaching, I wasn't good. No one is good when they are learning Jimmy.

HOPE WITHIN ME

You will learn as you grow. When I first started teaching at my first school, I was awful. My students made fun of me." He laughed.

I was crying, but his comment had made me laugh a bit too. Dr. Marino's arm was around my shoulder, which comforted me to an extent.

"For you, I would look out of your score. Know your music and make eye contact with them. That's where you should start. We all start somewhere. And most importantly, have fun." He finished with a smile, which cheered me up.

We both went back inside to regroup for the end of the rehearsal.

. . . . .

October went well that year, and since the talk with Dr. Marino, I started to feel optimistic about the children's choir. And everything with the music fraternity, that I had been initiated into back in the spring of 2016, had been going great too. Events were on rare occasions and weekly meetings were only to brief the chapter on what was going on throughout the week or month. Classes, opera rehearsals, children's choir, and the fraternity had seemed to be going great.

SUNDAY, NOVEMBER 20, 2016

It was the day of the children's choir concert. The professors and the four of us choral music education students were preparing for the concert. Excited, we got the children lined up, as we watched the parents and even our own parents sat in the audience. My peers were conducting before me. There were four pieces of music before it was time for my turn to conduct. I walked onto the stage and gestured towards the pianist so we could bow together.

I smiled at the children; some had smiled back. I raised my hands and made eye contact with the pianist. I took a deep breathe with the children and mouthed the words with them and they were singing. I couldn't believe it, words came out of their mouths, with me in front of them conducting. Halfway through the piece, I started to notice something wasn't right. I had lost track of where I was. I was a page behind where the children and pianist were. Luckily, the pianist had noticed I had lost track, so she had started to play the children's part on the piano while I tried to find my place. I kept conducting, so no one in the audience noticed only Dr. Anders and Dr. Marino did. Confused and sad at how I had lost time and music with the children during the performance, I gestured to the children, and had them bow. I then gestured to the pianist and bowed with her and mouthed *Thank You* to her before I walked off the stage.

. . . . .

The following school day, I had been asked to come into the front office to speak to Dr. Anders and Dr. Marino.

"Good afternoon Jimmy. We wanted to congratulate you on a wonderful children's choir concert yesterday." Dr. Anders started by saying.

"But Dr. Marino and I noticed something unusual about your conducting during the performance that we had never seen during the rehearsals" She said.

" We noticed you were behind a significant amount, and you looked a little strange while conducting. No one in the audience noticed, but we did." Dr. Marino added.

"Yeah, I noticed I was behind almost a whole page. I don't know how though. At first I thought the children had slowed down, or maybe the piano did. So, I quickly tried to find where they were. Luckily, the pianist doubled their part for me until I found the right page."

"We're not doctors, but do you think it was possible, without you knowing, that you had a seizure while you were conducting?" Dr. Anders asked.

"It's possible. Though I didn't feel the normal aura or anything. I did feel strange up there though. And the fact that I lost over five to ten seconds worth of music was scary." I told them both, as I tried to figure out why I had lost time in the music during my conducting.

"Yeah, that's pretty scary stuff. Maybe it was and you didn't know it?" Dr. Marino said.

"Okay, well that's all we wanted to know. We just wanted to make sure you were feeling okay because we had never seen you act like that while conducting." Dr. Anders said as we finished the meeting.

Many years later, I would come to realize that it was actually a Focal Onset Aware Seizure that had occurred during that performance.

.　.　.　.　.

By December, I had made the decision to discontinue to be one of the conductors of the children's choir as I had been afraid of having too much stress and causing an actual seizure. Though, years later I would come to learn it was one. The spring I would focus on classes, the opera role, choir, and the fraternity.

FRATERNITY ELECTIONS - SPRING 2017

It was January, and Christmas break had ended. The second semester had started, and I was no longer a conductor of the children's choir, which I felt guilty about, but was more concerned about my health and classes so I also felt relieved as well. The semester was filled with opera rehearsals for the production taking place in March, choir rehearsals, and fraternity events.

By the second semester, everyone in the opera and with lead roles were to be off score and have their roles memorized. That wasn't the case for certain members, as even my counterpart, as we had all been double casted, didn't know his music or French yet. The rehearsals were interesting, as the only thing that kept us sane and having fun was interacting with each other. So, Professor Mark, the Opera Director, adjusted the schedule. It would be a long road to production.

Come February, the fraternity announced they would be holding elections for new

officers for the following year. My friend Kris and I had started to think about running for an

office in the fraternity. Throughout the beginning of February, I had worked with the Vice

President to host *Music Appreciation Week*, so I had started to want his position. My friend Kris

had started to talk with the President to get to know his position. Kris and I were almost certain

we knew what we wanted but still trying to decide.

It was the end of February, and time for nominations. Kris and I, along with other

members, were both nominated for Vice President and President. I knew what I wanted, so I

declined the President nomination and accepted the Vice President one. We were told to have our

speeches prepared for the positions for election night in March.

On March 21, 2017, the fraternity held the elections for the offices of President and Vice

President. Kris and myself both hoped he would get President and I Vice President. The chapter

sent him and others outside of the room, and it only took minutes before they were let back into

the room before they announced Kris the new President for 2017-2018 school year.

I was sent out next, along with the candidates who had lost to Kris for President. They

had decided to run for Vice President. We stood outside, with our ears against the door to try and

hear if we could make out their conversation about one of us. It took fifteen minutes before they

came to let us in. We had all sat down, when someone stood up in the center of the room, as he

did for Kris, and announced, "The new Vice President of the fraternity for the 2017-2018 school year is Jimmy Valencia!".

I couldn't believe my ears at the time. I had been able to beat the opponents who had run for President against Kris and also tried to run for Vice President. I was happier than could be. The weeks that followed, Kris and I met with the current brothers who held those offices to receive tips and for them to pass along knowledge of the fraternity.

THE OPERA - MARCH 31, 2017

After many weeks of rehearsals, it was opening night for the opera! I had been rehearsing the

lead role I was given, the prior spring of 2016, and had worked on the pronunciation of the

French with my private voice instructor as well as with Professor Mark. It would soon be time to

open the show at seven o'clock in the evening on Friday, March 31. My counterpart, who didn't

know the part as well as I did, would perform the second night, April 1, so I was given opening

night. As the lights went dark, the performance began, with the orchestra softly playing the

Entr'acte.

It was three thirds through the opera where I had my lead role, and I felt great. Feeling

the French role off my tongue, a language I was not fond of, in front of hundreds of audience

members. It was an exhilarating experience that I had never felt before. It would be halfway into a half spoken, half sung line when I felt the feeling. The aura and warning. I thought I would be able to sing through it. Dr. Anders came running up the side of stage right to the backstage.

The orchestra played a sustained note, while the conductor waited to cue me, wondering why I hadn't started my new line, as I stood there, not able to sing, frozen. My counterpart, knowing what was happening and being across the stage, came out and sang the rest of the line. It gave the conductor time to cue the orchestra to play the rest of the part. Dr. Anders opened the stage right door and gently called me to come. I walked off stage, still coming out of the seizure, and sat in a chair with Dr. Anders.

Embarrassed, not believing what had happened in front of all of the audience members, I started to realize it.

"Jimmy, are you okay?" Dr. Anders asked.

"Yeah, I'm fine now."

Ten minutes later, someone came to Dr. Anders and asked if I could finish my role, as the *Finale* approached.

"We don't know yet." She told them.

"Do you think you can go back out there? You don't have to if you can't. Your counterpart can do it." She looked at me, waiting for a response.

I had spent an entire year memorizing, working on pronunciation of French, and leaning music. I needed to get my Finale. I can't let my Epilepsy ruin this for me. I thought to myself

"Yeah, I can finish it." I told her.

" Are you positive Jimmy?" She asked again, not believing me.

"Yeah." I said as I stood up and headed to the stage door.

I waited and listened to the orchestra. I knew when the cue for the *Finale* was. So, as soon as it was time, I let myself out the door and onto the stage.

It was time, so I had let myself onto the stage.

"Voila!" I had sang.

The conductor, stared at me, shocked I came back onto the stage to finish. My counterpart quickly left the stage on the other side with the stage left door. I finished the opera *Finale* dramatically as planned, with the spotlight on me, as I fell to my knees center stage, hands in my face before the lights faded and the orchestra finished playing. At the end, the cast came out to meet me on stage, the lights turned up, and we all bowed together.

At the end of the opera, as much of a disappointment as it was, the audience hadn't noticed the seizure. It had all looked like it was a part of the production, the way I had walked off stage and my counterpart took over for me. Only for me to return later to end the *Finale*.

. . . . .

It was soon the end of junior year. I had been placed in *Mixed Auditioned Singers*, became the Vice President of the fraternity and had performed in an opera production. It had been a successful year. Disappointed in the seizure incident at the opera, but happy no one noticed except the performers, my family and myself.

The end of junior year only got better though because in the coming summer, I was studying abroad in Austria. I would be studying *Classical Music Literature* with Dr. Bailey in Salzburg, Austria.

STUDY ABROAD – SUMMER 2017

Before I went abroad to Europe, I met with Doctor Klark. We went over how I had been feeling and been doing with my seizures. Although I was still having them frequently, it was manageable. My reason for the visit that day was to get a month and a half's worth of medication, which needed to be approved. So, I told him of my study of abroad and he wished me luck and to just track anything while I was out in Europe.

It was the day after my twenty first birthday, as my family and I had celebrated it early and I had packed for my Study Abroad in Salzburg, Austria. I was headed to the airport in Los Angeles ready for my first international flight. The program I was enrolled in was from June 4 – 27, but it would take a day to get to Europe, so I had booked a ticket earlier than that. We had arrived at the airport at six o'clock in the evening when I ran into friends who were also taking

JAMES VALENCIA

the *Classical Music Literature* Study Abroad course. I said my farewells to my parents and sisters before I went up the escalators to the security checkpoint with my friends.

I talked to a friend who was also nervous but excited to go and study in a country where classical music was birthed. We waited in the security checkpoint line when I felt the sensation go through my body. I had ignored it at first, and it had seemed to go away. But, a minute later, I felt the sensation again, and the next thing I came to realize was that I was sitting on a stool in the security checkpoint line with my friend who was standing next to me. She knew I had Epilepsy and had seen my seizures before, so she knew what to do. The airport security officers had offered a stool for me to sit on until I was okay. Security flagged my ticket so they could come and check on me before boarding, though they never did. Embarrassed, with all the passengers who passed me trying to get through security, my friend stayed with me the entire time. I kept apologizing, but she told me not to worry.

We continued to the gate, where we waited a few hours, as we had a red eye to Philadelphia. There, we waited ten hours before a nine-hour flight into Munich. When we had arrived in Munich, we took a two-hour train ride to Salzburg and finally arrived at our housing at noon on June 4. Dr. Bailey, who was teaching the course, met us at the front door to give us our room assignments. I was rooming with Kris and Ted, both from the fraternity. After a day of travelling, I was happy to see Kris and Ted, and to just rest.

Dr. Bailey pulled me aside during dinner that evening to talk to me privately. I had been scared my friend had told her about the incident at the airport back in the United States.

"Jimmy, I wanted to give you this lift pass." Dr. Bailey handed me a pass.

"There is a giant elevator that you can use." She told me.

The housing we stayed at was located on a giant mountain that overlooked Salzburg. And to go back and forth between the city and the house involved a lot of stairs.

"As you know, we are up on a mountain, and going up and down the mountain can be very strenuous. With your Epilepsy I want to make sure you don't have any problems while you're studying here. The pass is good for thirty days and for two people, so you can use it for yourself and another person, like a friend." She told me.

"Okay, thank you Dr. Bailey. How much was it; I can pay you back for it?" I asked her.

I had felt bad she went out of her way to buy the pass, as the thirty-day pass wasn't cheap.

"Don't worry about paying me back for it, I just want to make sure you are okay while you are here studying and going back and forth between the house and Salzburg."

"Thank you so much Dr. Bailey." I said with a smile before we both left.

I went back to the room to find Kris and Ted. We sat and planned our weekend trips. The weekends were the only days we didn't have class and travelled. The first weekend, Friday June 9 – Sunday June 11, the whole class went to Vienna. There, we took a tour of the Wiener Staatsoper (Vienna Opera House), saw and listened to Wiener Philharmoniker (the Vienna

Philharmonic) and went to the Wiener Hofmusikkapelle where we listened to Mozart's *Missa Brevis, B-Dur,* KV 275.

The second weekend, Saturday June 17 – Monday June 19, Kris, Ted, and I headed to Prague. We went to clubs and an Ice Pub. And the third weekend, Thursday June 22 – June Monday 26, the three of us went to Paris where we saw the Mona Lisa at the Louvre, went to the Eiffel Tower every night and visited the Arc de Triomphe.

. . . . .

The month of the Study Abroad in Salzburg and Classical Music with Dr. Bailey went by quick, but we had learned so much about the culture of Europe and music. We had also gotten the chance to travel throughout the continent with each other, have fun, and make memories. Although I had a seizure on the first day at the airport, I had been seizure free the rest of the month, and it felt good.

On Wednesday June 28, it was time to head home for everyone. Most of us had been booked on the same flight, so at four o'clock in the morning, we said our good-byes to Dr. Bailey, and headed to the train station and airport together. We departed Munich once again, only to land in London, this time with a two-hour layover and prepared for our twelve-hour flight to Los Angeles. There, we all said our farewells to each other for the rest of Summer.

136

FALL 2017

It was SENIOR YEAR OF COLLEGE. The four years of undergrad had gone by quickly for me. At that point, I had been living with Epilepsy for more than seven years. But, I had made great friends, was in an uplifting fraternity that I was the Vice President of and had mentors who were willing to help me in any situation. I had only met with my neurologist a few times over the past four years and I was still having seizures, but I felt safe in the environment I was in at the college though. I looked forward to what that academic year would bring my friends and myself.

As any of the years started, auditions were held. I was again placed in *Mixed Auditioned Singers*. The group that year was special, because we were to travel to an international conference to perform the following summer in 2018. So, Dr. Anders and Dr. Marino made the audition process hard that year. The members in the ensemble were also given hard and fun music, but Dr. Anders taught it slow and in fun ways, which made it less stressful.

It was fun being the Vice President of the fraternity I was in, especially with my friend Kris. We planned many events for the School of Music and college, fundraisers, and even a retreat for the fraternity so we could bond as a group. Kris and I worked well together, and we often stayed late at the college on occasion to plan things for meetings and events. So, our friend Ted, who was our roommate in Salzburg and also in the fraternity, would let me stay over at his apartment during the week on some nights when I needed it. This meant I carried an extra set of clothes and toothbrush in my backpack on certain days.

It was nice that Ted let me stay the night every so often, or as he said, "whenever you need or want Jimmy". It came in handy for me because I used to ride my bicycle to school, until one day that fall, I came out of class and it was gone. Someone had stolen my bicycle, or at least everything except the front tire that was still locked up. My bicycle was a road bicycle, it was over $1,200, and I was not happy. Eventually, my mother heard of a ridesharing service and I started to use that. She told me she would pay for it. I was hesitant at first, but it worked for the time being. I felt bad using her credit card every day, as it was $20 a day. So, I created my own account and attached my credit card to it instead. But, to cut back on the cost, I started to spend the night at Ted's place more often which ended up being fun for us, and even all of our friends that would come over and hangout too.

HOPE WITHIN ME

Senior year of college was stressful, and I was having multiple seizures that year. I was having one or two seizures every two weeks. The combination of classes, choir, private lessons, the fraternity meetings, and just daily life stressed me out. To me, a seizure every week or two had become normal. It wasn't though, and it never should have become normal to me. In November, Dr. Anders gave me an offer, one that I almost took.

"Jimmy, can I speak to you outside please?" she asked me in the hallway.

"Uh...sure." I replied. We both walked out to the patio of the School of Music.

"You've been having quite a few seizures the past couple of months. The Christmas Performance is coming up in a couple of weeks, and I want to let you make the decision if you want or do not want to perform in it. For your mental health and physical health."

My grade in Mixed Auditioned Singers though. It will go down by 50% for missing a performance! That was all I could think of right after she said that to me. But almost as if she had read my mind, staring into my eyes and knew what I had thought she said,

"And it will not impact your grade in *Mixed Auditioned Singers* whatsoever. I am the Director of the Christmas Performance, so I can excuse anyone I want. As of right now, you have 100% in my ensemble for the semester. Let me know what you think, okay Jimmy?"

"Okay Dr. Anders, thank you." I replied. She smiled and we both walked back inside the building.

That was all I could think about the rest of that day. Did I want to perform, or not? I always had seizures and was stressed during that time of the year. But, it was my Senior year of college, and the Christmas performance had meant so much to me. And knowing how much Dr. Anders trusted me by letting me know I had a good grade in her ensemble meant a lot. It was emotional trying to decide. At the next rehearsal I had made my decision. I went to her and let her know I wanted to perform and knew I could. When the Christmas Performance came a couple weeks later, it was one of the most memorable. It was my last one as an undergraduate student, and I had no issues with seizures during the rehearsals or performances. It had all gone smoothly, and I was glad I had chosen to perform instead of living in my fear of having a seizure. The semester had ended, and I couldn't believe I was halfway done with Senior year.

. . . . .

In December, it was time for another appointment with Doctor Klark. The last time I had seen him was before I had gone abroad to Salzburg. I sat down, and we started with how my trip abroad went. Then, I proceeded to tell him about the seizure I had in the airport. I also told him of the other seizures throughout the fall. Again, no reaction from him though. He insisted there had been no change or digression with my Epilepsy. He told me that a seizure every two weeks was normal for someone with my diagnosis. So, it was a short appointment. We shook hands and I left.

HOPE WITHIN ME

No one should believe that multiple seizures a week is normal, but I had been told that for years. Drilled into my head as a belief that it was normal, so I had started to believe it. That it was the way my life was going to be forever.

SENIOR RECITAL - WEDNESDAY MARCH 21, 2018

Senior year of college continued, and it was spring and time for my senior recital. I would be singing an hours' worth of music for that recital since I was a double major in music. Throughout that day, I was stressed more than ever. I had been trying to remember words to songs as most of them were in other languages, notes, dynamics, everything. I was also excited though because I knew most of my friends were going to be there, as well as my family. The recital wasn't until six o' clock that evening, so I had plenty of time to relax and warmup at home before I had to arrive at the recital hall.

It was nearing four o' clock, so I had already headed to the School of Music to get comfortable in the recital hall where I was going to be performing. I ran through a couple spots in each of my pieces with the pianist I was collaborating with and rested until the doors opened. I waited backstage until six o' clock. I peeked out into the audience a couple of times amazed at how many people had shown up, surprised that even Dr. Anders had shown up. It was the same recital hall I had auditioned in, only it was filled with around sixty-five to seventy people. My voice professor came backstage to calm my nerves and ask if I was ready to perform. Before I knew it, I was walking out onto the stage with giant spotlights shining on me.

As the pieces went by that night, my confidence grew. I was pleased with how well I sounded and was performing in front of everyone. I walked backstage to rest before the last piece. With no aura or warning, not even a feeling, I fell. The pianist helped me sit on a chair backstage. There had been a loud sound that came from the backstage area, so my voice professor came to see what happened. My mother followed, only to assume that I had a seizure. As the seizure came to an end, I was eager to get back out and finish the recital. The pianist asked if I wanted to use music for the last piece, but I had insisted I didn't need it.

I walked back out onto the stage for the last piece, excited but more scared not to mess up, as I had worked tirelessly on that piece from *Ragtime*. I nodded to the pianist so we could get started. I only got through one verse before I stopped singing. I didn't remember the words. I stared at the back of the recital hall as I tried to remember but couldn't. The pianist quickly handed me the book, and we started where we had left off. I was embarrassed, I had never forgotten words before. As soon as the piece ended, I bowed and quickly walked backstage. My voice teacher came and asked me to go back out and bow again even though I didn't want to.

After the recital, there was a reception for the guests and me. I waited to go, as I went to the bathroom and cried for a while. I was embarrassed, as I had worked so hard, and it felt like it had been stolen from me in a matter of seconds because of something I wasn't able to control. I sat in the private bathroom for a few minutes before I knew I had to go to the reception. My parents had spent so much time and money putting it together for me, and I needed to thank everyone who had come. It was the most depressing reception I had been to in all my years of recitals, as I fought back tears and anger. As soon as I arrived home with my parents, I went upstairs and cried. I cried out to God, to myself, and was angry at myself for the way I was.

The following day I had *Mixed Auditioned Singers*, I was still depressed from the day before, but Dr. Anders had mentioned how well I had sang in the recital in front of the entire ensemble. It made me happy for a while before the thought of how my Epilepsy had ruined the last piece of the recital. But I was glad she enjoyed it, and others did too. It was hard to think about that recital the rest of that year.

. . . . .

I had booked my recital at the end of the semester, so the rest of that year went by fast.

It was time for graduation! I couldn't believe it, after all the hard work I had put into all of my music and non-music courses for four years. And after four years of professors, friends, fraternity, and family who had supported and uplifted me throughout my time at the small Liberal Arts College and helped support me with my health, it was time to leave. It was going to be a hard transition, but I knew I was going to be able to do it. All that was left to do was go on the choir trip with *Mixed Auditioned Singers*, which we eventually did in July of 2018 after graduation.

The day had arrived, Friday April 20, 2018. The day of graduation went by fast and it was a surreal day to me. I started the day with morning mimosas at the fraternity house with friends before I headed back home to get ready. It was filled with emotions, good and bad memories, and laughter with friends. I will never forget how the Chancellor mentioned my name in his speech he addressed to the graduating class, I don't think my mother will either. The day ended, and there I was, a college graduate with a degree. I did it! Little did I know what lay ahead of me was greater. A greater battle, but a greater hope.

III

.....

III

PLAN FOR GRADUATE SCHOOL

It was the summer after I had graduated from my undergraduate when I decided to apply for a Master's in Education. It was the best decision, as I was already Student-Teaching in the coming fall, and it would help cover the cost of tuition. So, I had applied again to the Liberal Arts College and was accepted. I started graduate classes and Student-Teaching at a high school that fall. I taught multiple music courses which included, Beginning Choir, Advanced Choir, and A.P. Music Theory. I was overseen by the actual teacher of the classroom, Steven, my master teacher for the semester. He evaluated me throughout my time at the high school.

My largest concern was the possibility of having a seizure during Student-Teaching. I was hesitant to let Steven know the first day, as we had just met, but he was a laid-back person. So, on the second day, I let him know about my Epilepsy. He wasn't concerned about it, he just wanted to know how he could help and what to do. That made me happy, and confident in Steven. He ended up being a reliable master teacher throughout that semester. After the many graduate school night classes, even though they were once a week, and teaching five days for seven hours a day every week, the semester had finished. It was sad to say good-bye to the students at the high school. I had realized first-hand the bond I had built with them.

I had also realized one other thing, from September through December I had absolutely no seizures. For the first time in years, I had gone months seizure free! *Could this have been it? Could this have been the very thing I had been waiting for since I was fourteen years old, now that I was twenty-two?* After I had departed the high school for the last time that fall in 2018, I was ready to finish the Master's of Education program in the coming spring. Things had started to look up.

In mid-January, I received my preliminary teaching credential for the state of California in music education. I couldn't have been more excited. All that was left to do that semester was to finish the Master's program. For the program, I only had to take one more course, a writing seminar for the twenty-five to thirty-page thesis. I had finished most of the courses in my undergraduate studies, as I had taken graduate level education classes.

As the new and last semester began that January, things had felt good, and I felt confident that it was all going well until the month of February came. I had the first seizure since the fall in early September of 2018. It broke my heart, months of being seizure free was gone in just a blink of an eye. I tried to reassure myself a "breakthrough" seizure was going to occur every so often, so I tried to keep my head up. Except, only over the next few days more seizures followed. Every two weeks I had a seizure, then it turned into every week. It became a constant rate of seizures that spring of 2019, every week, then every other week.

. . . . .

By the middle of March, it was time for my appointment with Doctor Klark. I desperately wanted answers. *Why were my seizure getting worse? Was it stress? Is it normal?* I met with Dr. Klark that spring and showed him the journal of all the seizure activity that had occurred over the past couple of months. He was shocked.

"Has anything changed, like lifestyle, stress, etc." he asked me.

"I am stressed over school, but that's normal. Nothing else." I told him. He wrote it down like he always did.

"I want to increase your *Oxcarbazepine*." He said.

Thank God, an answer!

"You're taking 2 600mg tab/2x daily right now, right?"

" Yeah, I am."

"Starting tonight, I want you to take 2 ½ 600mg tab/2x daily."

"Okay." I replied, hoping that the increased dosage was going to solve my problems.

"I think we are all good here James." He stood up, shook my hand, and walked out.

As I left the room, I felt confident all would work out. And it seemed as if it did. The seizures started to slow down for a while. Instead of every week, every two weeks, to every three weeks. And it had stayed that way, but I was content living life that way because as sad as it was, it became all I knew.

.   .   .   .

I finally started to finish writing the thesis that would complete the Master's I had worked hard on, and graduation day was upon me again. On Thursday April 25, 2019, I graduated with the Master's in Education. It wasn't as exciting as the undergraduate graduation, but I felt more accomplished than the previous year. It was a great evening; I went to dinner with my parents and sisters and it was great to see how proud my parents were of me. I knew I had to start looking for jobs though, so the following day, I started to apply for music positions. I started to get worried though, as it would soon be May, and then June and I still had no reply from any school district on job offers. I had been interviewed multiple times, but not contacted.

It was early July 2019 when I received an offer for a position. It was a position for an elementary choir teacher. If I accepted the job, I was to teach first through sixth grade classes and need to create a curriculum in less than a month. I decided to take the offer, I knew at that moment I needed to start somewhere, and elementary sounded fun. I had taught the children's choir back in college, although it was only for a semester. As I planned the curriculum, and had set everything up, I started to get nervous about my Epilepsy. What if I had a seizure in front of the children. I had been having seizures every three weeks, so I just hoped it wasn't going to happen while I taught.

In mid-July, the seizure activity started to increase again. I tried to ignore it as I wanted to think it would stop. But it had soon gone from every two weeks to every week again. I started to get nervous and frustrated at that point because I had to start teaching in only a matter of weeks. So, I set up an appointment with Doctor Klark. When I met with him that time, his plan of action was almost immediate.

"I want to try this clinical trial drug that may work for you. It's called, *Lamotrigine*. Here are the instructions." He wrote them on a piece of yellow paper and handed it to me and read:

"Take 25mg:

1 tab/2x daily for 2 weeks

Then,

2 tab/2x daily for 2 weeks

Then,

Take 100mg 2x/daily.

Call if seizures continue and dose can be increased or if a rash form." All of this read aloud to me and handed to me on paper.

Doctor Klark and I walked to a closet where he pulled out bottles of Anti-Epileptic Drugs (AEDs) and handed me a couple of them.

"They don't have these at pharmacies yet, so when and if you need more call and we can get you more." He told me before he walked me out.

Excited about the new medication I had received, I started it that evening. But within just days, I started to get bumps on my feet. I kept taking the medication for a few more days before I finally called the neurology office and told them about the rash. Once again, I was at an appointment with Doctor Klark.

"Hello James, let's take a look at your rash." He looked over my feet.

"Yeah, that's from the *Lamotrigine*. I have another medication that may work better for you instead of the *Lamotrigine*. I want you to start taking this new medication called *Lacosamide*. This one is not a clinical trial and is an anticonvulsant. I want you to take 1 200mg tab/2x daily."

"Okay." I replied, happy to stop the *Lamotrigine*.

Later that evening I went to the pharmacy to pick up the new medication and started the dosage Doctor Klark had told me to take.

With all the seizures I had, I started to think I needed a specialist again. I needed an adult

HOPE WITHIN ME

Epileptologist, someone who specialized in Epilepsy and seizures only. So, I started the long journey and fight with the insurance company to get myself into the *Medical Center* I had first started with when I was a teenager. I knew I needed to do *something*, as my seizures had gotten worse. I needed to think about the future. I was getting ready for a career and needed it under control.

157

MY CAREER BEGINS

It was August 2019 when I started to teach at the elementary school. I was nervous, but excited to finally put my degrees to use. It had felt weird to be in charge of my own classroom full of students looking at me. I had no master teacher, or professors to guide me, it was just myself and it felt great. The first two weeks of teaching choir had gone smoothly, with the children learning the music quite well. Other than a few seizures at home every so often, things were good, and I had finally felt confident in myself.

In the middle of August, I decided to join a professional choral ensemble so I could keep my voice up while I taught. I auditioned for the *Master Chorale Singers*. I ended up being accepted into the group and rehearsed on Tuesday evenings after I was done teaching. It was great, a member of the choir was the choir director of the high school near where I taught.

Aside from being in *Master Chorale Singers* and rehearsal, teaching went well until September came. It happened out of nowhere, I felt the feeling. I tried to push it away knowing I couldn't. I had a seizure in front of my students. A teacher aide was in the room and was able to call the nurse and homeroom teachers. I had never felt more embarrassed, as I had just started my career and within the first month I had a seizure. The school district nurse and my supervisor wanted to speak to me that day, so choir was cancelled the rest of the day, which made me worried about falling behind in lessons, which should have been the least of my concern.

"Good morning James how are you feeling?" the district nurse asked.

"I feel fine." I told her. Part of me wanted to cry, but more so I felt the shame I used to feel when I started back at the college, back when no one knew of this part of me that I wish never existed.

"So today you had a seizure?" she asked. Both her and my supervisor looked at me.

"Yes. I take medication for it. It usually controls it though."

"Would you think it would be helpful if we made an action plan in case something like this happens again? Would you be comfortable with that?" My supervisor asked.

"I'd appreciate that." I told her.

The three of us sat there and talked about my seizures and Epilepsy. I told them both how I had lived with Epilepsy for over nine years and had been on and off medications. I explained what to do and what not to do if I had another seizure in front of the classroom. We sat there as the nurse typed up a *Seizure Emergency Action Plan*. The final copy read:

IF YOU SEE THIS:

    Seizure Type: *Impaired Awareness Seizure*

    Seizure Appearance: *Staring off, zoning out, loss of time*

    Triggers to Start a Seizure: *Stress, tired*

    Usual Length of Seizure: *30-60 seconds*

    Medication: *Oxcarbazepine (2.5 tabs-600mg each) and Lacosamide (1 tab-200mg each)*

    Last Seizure: *September 2019*

DO THIS:

- *Protect individual from injury*

- *Do **NOT** attempt to move the individual during the seizure*

- *Monitor the individual until he regains full consciousness*

- *Protect individual's head from hitting the ground*

- *Do **NOT** put anything in the individual's mouth*

- *Notify the school nurse and individual's emergency contact*

- *As soon as possible, turn individual on his side in the recovery position in case of vomiting. Keep in this position until he regains consciousness*

- *Stay calm and reassuring*

- *Time and document seizure activity*

JAMES VALENCIA

CALL 911 IF:

- *Absence of breathing and/or pulse*
- ***Seizure- 2 minutes or longer***
- *A tonic clonic seizure (this is atypical as he has never had a tonic clonic)*
- *Two or more consecutive seizures (without a period of consciousness between)*

INDIVIDUAL ADAPTIONS:

*James has had seizures since 2010 and takes daily medication. Prior to having a seizure he may experience an aura. If James is able, he will hold up 1 finger to alert staff and take a seat in the chair that he will keep next to him. A staff member should stay near James and assist him as needed while following the above seizure guidelines. James' seizures typically last 30-60 seconds. Please time the seizure. **If the seizure lasts longer than 2 minutes or he experiences a tonic clonic seizure please call 911.** While one staff member is with James, the other staff members should escort the students back to class. After the seizure has passed, please escort him to the health office and allow him to rest (it is more comfortable for him to sit). Please do not offer water unless James requests it. While he is resting in the health office, please contact his father **first** to come pick him up. If unable to reach his father, contact his mother. If his mother is unavailable contact his grandfather. All emergency numbers are attached. Please notify the district nurse.*

Seizure Emergency Action Plan completed by District School Nurse.

162

HOPE WITHIN ME

After she had printed a copy for me to take home, she put it in a maroon folder that read "Confidential". They wished me well, and I headed home to change lesson plans for the following day. The rest of the week went by smoothly, and all I looked forward to was *Master Chorale Singers* rehearsal. Singing in choir was all that brought joy to me that week and the following weeks. Until I stood in front of my first graders one day in September and felt it again. The aura, the rising sensation in my body I had grown accustomed to for so many years. But there was a plan that time. I saw the chair to the side of the piano where I had put it before I had started class. Still talking to the kids, I walked to the chair slowly. I raised one finger in the air to notify the teacher aide, and I sat down in the chair. In a matter of a minute, the seizure was over and there were homeroom teachers in my classroom. Some escorted the children back to their room, and a few stayed with me. Once again I journeyed back to the health office. That shameful walk, I felt the eyes of all the secretaries stare at me. I could only imagine what they thought of me, *a teacher, going to the health office*? The problem was that wasn't the last time I made that walk or the last seizure I had in front of my students. I had a total of five seizures before I called Dr. Klark and requested and MRI. To my surprise, he agreed, a fresh MRI sounded like a good idea to him. So, on Thursday October 3, I was scheduled for an MRI. I emailed my supervisor to let her know I needed the day off for it. Hours later I received a reply from my supervisor, who approved the day off, but also wanted to speak to me at the district office. *This was it. I'm getting fired, I just know it. My first job, no letter of recommendation, nothing.*

Thursday October 3, 2019 I went to my MRI appointment. It went by fast, as I had done multiple before. The sound of the buzzing machine, the fitted cage around my head, all so familiar. I was in and out in less than an hour. The real nerve wrecking thing on my mind was the meeting I was to have at the district office the next day.

I met with my supervisor along with the director of H.R. on Friday October 4, 2019. Terrified, not fully knowing what was to come, I sat in the lobby of the district office and waited for my supervisor that morning.

"Good morning James." my supervisor greeted me.

"Good morning." I tried not to look too scared.

"I've asked the director of H.R. to sit in with us as well, as she would like to explain some stuff."

"Okay." We had entered the H.R. director's office where there were three seats for us.

"Hello James, I'm the director of H.R."

"Hello." I smiled and shook her hand.

"So, James I want to let you know how great you are doing with the children and how they love the music." My supervisor started by saying. "But the school and I are starting to get concerned about your seizures in front of the children."

There it was, the judgement, the shame, it had all come back. Something I thought I had escaped. Nowhere to hide, exposed for something I can't control.

"We think it would be best if we discontinue choir and music for the time being."

"Okay." I replied.

"We want you to know how grateful we are for you, and that we are doing this because we think you should take the time to focus on your health. We would not have hired you if you were not qualified, which you certainly are." She continued.

I fought back every emotion within myself.

"Also, even though you aren't going to be physically working, we want to keep paying you through your contract." the H.R. director told me.

"Oh, okay. Thank you." I said, shocked. Although, I did not know at that time they legally were required to since I had filled out the accommodation form for my Epilepsy.

The meeting ended with a few handshakes before I left the district office. I was angry, embarrassed, ashamed for the part of me I wasn't able to control. I tried to look on the bright side though, I was still getting paid, and didn't need to work. Luckily, I used the rest of October to plan my mother's birthday celebration. So, I was able to take my mind off of my health for a while and enjoyed life as much as I was able to, which was a difficult task to do at the time.

FRIENDS - WEDNESDAY NOVEMBER 6, 2019

I was headed to Los Angeles with friends, and it was going to be a great day. We stopped for coffee before we left, and blared music out the windows on the freeway. We were talking and laughing, but I didn't feel good. My friends had noticed too, but before I knew it, I had gone into a seizure. But not long after the first, came another seizure.

"Jimmy are you okay?" they asked me.

"Yeah, I feel fine now."

"You had two seizures back-to-back."

"Really? I only remember the one. What happened?" I asked. I couldn't remember the second seizure at all. I had remembered the aura for the first seizure, but not the second.

"You tried to open the car door on the freeway, so we had to get off the freeway."

"Oh wow. I've never done that before." I replied.

"Yeah, we had to pull you away from the door."

After I had gotten the details about the two seizures, we stopped for more coffee, as I was trying to enjoy my time. Sometime later, we ended up at a random mall in Los Angeles, and we all walked around and looked at random stores. I started to get happy again, and even started to laugh and joke with my friends. But, again, I felt it. That rising sensation, I couldn't stop it. I tried to sit down on the floor by a wall in the mall, but it was too late. My friends stayed with me until it was over. I stood up, shook it off and we went about the mall. I wasn't going to let my emotions get to me, even if I wanted to cry, I held it in, I knew I had to be strong.

I saw a candle store while we had been walking earlier, so a friend who also loved candles went with me to look around. I figured since I was a huge candle person, the candle store would cheer me up a bit, along with some sarcasm from my friend and myself. We each bought their overpriced candles, but as we walked out of the store, the feeling returned. Immediately, I handed my bad to my friend and told her I needed to sit down. She helped me sit down right outside of the candle store. As soon as I came out of the seizure, I saw people staring, but my friend was sitting next me as she waited for me to be okay.

"Are you okay?" She asked.

"Yeah, I think I can get up now." I stood up with her help.

"You've had four seizures today." She told me

"Yeah, today has been weird."

"Do you want to go find the others? Maybe we can all get food now?" she asked.

Food sounded good at that point, as I had lost track of time and was hungry.

"Yeah, let's do it."

We went to find the others, as we were both hungry. When we all met up, we decided to eat somewhere on the way back home. So, we headed home and went through a drive thru. Music was back to blaring, and we had more coffee; I don't know what it was with our obsession with coffee, but we were laughing again. It was dusk and we were headed east towards our hometown when I felt the feeling again. Still forty minutes from home and on the freeway, I told my friends I was about to have a seizure. I ended up having the seizure, but when they explained the details to me, I wanted to cry not to expect what they would tell me.

"Jimmy are you sure you are okay right now?" they asked me, the driver still driving.

"Yeah, I'm just *extremely* tired. That felt like a really big seizure."

"No Jimmy. You just had three."

"I had three seizures?!" I didn't believe what I had just heard.

"Yeah. Like back-to-back, it was crazy. You came out of it, but in less than a minute you would have another. And you kept trying to open the car door." They explained.

"I'm so sorry." I felt nothing but shame, and embarrassment. "I know today was supposed to be fun, and I haven't made it that way." I told them.

"Don't even worry about it. And we did have fun! We had coffee, food, laughter, we're all here together. We just want to make sure you're okay. You had *seven seizures* total today. When you get home you really need to rest Jimmy." They reassured me.

"Yeah, I definitely just want to sleep."

They turned the music up and we started to talk and laugh again. In my head, I knew I needed to call Dr. Klark the next morning. As soon as I returned home, all of my friends hugged me, we said we loved each other, and I went up to my room before I laid down on my bed, sank into it, and fell asleep almost immediately.

. . . . . .

The following morning, Thursday November 7, I told my parents about the seizures from the previous day. I made a phone call to Doctor Klark as well and informed him that I had multiple seizures, some that I had not even been aware about. He immediately cleared one spot for me and scheduled me to come into his office at the earliest convenience that day. I went into see Doctor Klark that afternoon, and we talked about all of the seizures. We also talked about the findings from the MRI from October.

"Hello James, so you had multiple seizures yesterday?" Doctor Klark started by saying.

"Yes. I had seven in total."

"Tell what you can about them. Who was with you, and what you were doing?"

"Well, I was with a group of friends driving to Los Angeles and the first two seizures were in the car. They happened back-to-back, and I tried to open the car door, but my friends kept me from doing so." I told him as he took notes.

"What about the others?" He asked.

"I had two more in a mall we went to. One where I tried to sit down in the middle of the mall, but couldn't, so my friends helped guide me until it was over, and another with a friend near a candle store where I was able to sit down with her on the floor." I waited until he was done writing and thinking before I proceeded.

"Okay, that's four, that's a lot. What about the others?" He asked again.

"The last three happened in the car again, on the way back home from Los Angeles. It was the same as the first two. All three happened back to back, I didn't even know I had three, I thought it was one long seizure. And I tried to open the car door again, but my friends kept me from doing so." My hands trembled as I told him and at the thought of it.

"So, I've counted seven seizures. Many of them in clusters which is worrisome."

"I am actually trying to get into the *Medical Center* to see an adult Epileptologist, I'm just waiting for an appointment now in December." I told Doctor Klark.

"That's great to hear! A specialist will be able to help you more than I could, considering I am a general neurologist. I know about seizures, but an Epileptologist knows specifically about seizure disorders. I hope you can find an appointment soon."

"Yeah, I just need to wait now. But what do I do about the cluster of seizures. I didn't even know I had some of them yesterday?"

"I am going to prescribe you another medication on top of the others. It should help, it's called *Zonisamide*. I want you to take it in the evening or at bedtime with your evening medications. Here are the instructions, which I will write down for you.

Take:

1 100mg capsule/daily first week, 2 100mg capsules/daily second week,

3 100mg capsules/daily third week, 4 100mg capsules/daily fourth week.

I also want to go over your MRI findings before you leave." He told me.

"Oh, okay." I said, as he handed me the instructions then pulled out images of my brain.

"These are images of your brain from the MRI. I didn't find anything abnormal from the scan. There were a couple things that stood out but didn't raise any red flags. There was just some white substance which could be anything, nothing harmful, no tumor or anything."

"Are you sure it's nothing to worry about?"

"Yes, completely harmless, your MRI was perfectly fine. I've looked over many MRIs before and any neurologist would say the same."

"Okay." I didn't fully believe. I knew I needed to get into the *Medical Center*.

The Findings from October 3, 2019:

HOPE WITHIN ME

FINDINGS:

The ventricles are within normal limits in size. The

*midline structures appear intact. **A couple of rounded foci are seen***

overlying the left parietal lobe subcortical white matter measuring

***up to approximately 3 mm.** However, no cortical dysplasia or obvious*

heterotopia is seen. No diffusion restriction, intracranial

hemorrhage, mass effect, midline shift or abnormal contrast

enhancement is seen. There is mild mucosal thickening involving the

bilateral ethmoid air cells.

IMPRESSION:

A couple of 3 mm T2 hypertense foci are seen along the left parietal

***subcortical white matter, nonspecific.** Considerations would include*

possible vasculitis or possible association with migraines.

. . . . .

Since I had started a new medication, and had so many seizures in October and November, I decided I would take a "leave" from *Master Chorale Singers*. I wanted to focus on

173

JAMES VALENCIA

my health and make sure I didn't have any incidents during performances or rehearsals. It broke

my heart to leave the group for the rest of the fall and winter, but I told them I would be back in

the spring. The group was extremely supportive, as most of the members and the conductor knew

of my Epilepsy. To my surprise, the group sent me a card in the mail to wish me well, and how

they looked forward to seeing me in the spring. It was very heartwarming to know how

welcomed I was in the ensemble.

However, to focus on my health, I had one more obstacle to overcome, and it was to get

an appointment with an Epileptologist with the *Medical Center*.

IV

· · · · ·

A NEW DIAGNOSIS - DECEMEMBER 2019

It was December 16 when I had finally been able to schedule an appointment with the *Medical Center*. I had scheduled an appointment with Doctor Devrat, one of the top adult Epileptologist at the *Medical Center* (Not knowing he was at the time). I had gone with my father, who had driven me to the appointment.

"Hello James" Doctor Devrat shook my hand, then my father's. "So, you have a lot of seizures, can you describe them to me, what they look like, how long, feelings you have?"

"Well, I usually start by having an aura, but not all the time. It's like a fifty-fifty chance I'll have an aura before my seizure." I told him.

"Sometimes, has auras, sometimes doesn't" He said aloud while he wrote it down.

"Then, I start to stare into space or zone out. Maybe drool a little. I sometimes go on auto-pilot and start to walk around, or I'll try to automatically sit down wherever I'm at."

Doctor Devrat wrote *everything* down with detail, as he repeated every word I spoke aloud.

"Can you give me the dates of your last seizures within the last two months, and how many? He asked.

Yeah. I pulled out my seizure journal and read them, "October 8: one seizure, October 18: one seizure, October 29: one seizure, November 6: seven seizures."

"Seven seizures, November 6." I heard him write down and say out loud.

I continued, "November 29: one seizure, though I think that was from a fever, and December 11: one seizure. That was the last one I had." I closed the journal and set it down.

"They all seem to be a little more than a week a part. Can you tell me more about the November 6 seizures where you had seven? That's a lot for one day." Doctor Devrat asked.

I explained every detail I could, about the mall, and how my friends kept the car door closed on the freeway.

"From the information that I've gathered from you so far, it sounds like you have Focal Impaired Awareness Seizures. However, the cluster seizures you had back in November is worrisome as that can lead to more in the future, even Status Epilepticus."

"Okay." I didn't know what to say at the time.

"Overviewing your medication list, you are on quite a bit of AEDs. You are taking three of them, which is a lot, so I want to schedule you for bloodwork and routine labs for AED levels in your blood cells."

I just nodded, all of this sounded foreign to me.

"What this will tell me is how much of the medication is *actually* in your blood and if it is effective. It will also let me know if it is damaging your liver since you are on so many AEDs and high dosages." Doctor Devrat explained to my father and myself. I was happy he did.

"You have tried or been on five AEDs now, and your body hasn't seemed to respond to many of them."

"Yeah, the only one that has been the anchor for him has been the *Oxcarbazepine*, which he's been on since 2011 with Doctor Michaels back in Pediatric Neurology." My dad told him.

"Yeah, so when medications work and then fail for a patient, their body becomes immune to it. It's like when they take too much Tylenol or anything. But for Epilepsy patients, we call this Intractable Epilepsy, or Uncontrolled Epilepsy. Where no matter what AED we give them, it will work maybe for a week or month, but then stop working. We don't know why this happens. It happens to one in three people, and unfortunately, that is you. No matter what AED we give you, it will not work for long."

I sat in the chair in the doctor's office. I felt alone, scared, with my heart broken. I didn't know how to react other than to cry, but I held it in. I felt my throat tighten as I fought back the emotions and tears that wanted to form and scream out of my soul, out of my broken heart.

"James, have you looked into any other alternative options other than AEDs to help treat your seizures?" Doctor Devrat asked both my father and me.

I knew immediately what I wanted and needed. I was scared to even say it aloud, but I did because it had been part of the reason I wanted to go to the *Medical Center* as an adult.

"Yes, I am interested in surgery." My father knew I was going to mention it, but I saw out of the corner of my eye that he was just as nervous as I was.

"Epilepsy surgery is a great option, even devices implanted on the brain or removal of the part where the seizure activity is happening. Especially since your seizures are not well controlled. There is a process you will need to go through, as you will need to be a candidate. Let me give you a brief overview of the process, and again, no decision needs to be made anytime soon."

My father and I sat forward in our chairs and listened carefully as Doctor Devrat explained how the process would work.

"The risks and benefits need to be carefully discussed, which we did because your seizures are not controlled, as well as with the people going to perform the operation. There will also be certain testing that needs to be done, like MRIs, EEGs, Video EEGs, PET Scans and possibly more. All of this information I will review and present to a panel at the hospital and neurosurgeons and we will discuss whether you would be a good candidate for this type of operation."

My father and I just sat there and listened, shocked at how much needed to be done. We shouldn't have been shocked considering the operation though.

Doctor Devrat kept explaining the process, "The testing for candidacy can take anywhere from up to eight months to a year and a half at times. Also, having brain surgery does not guarantee that you will be seizure free or won't need to keep taking AEDs after the operation. Though chances are, you will either become seizure free afterwards or have less seizures while taking less AEDs." Doctor Devrat printed an incredibly detailed step by step process of how the candidacy process worked for my father and myself to take home that day.

"For now, before you leave today, here is a referral. I would like to see you back at the clinic in two months for a follow up. James, I want you to record any seizure activity you have. Also, I am sending a referral so you can have an outpatient EEG monitoring done in January." He walked out of the office to grab the referral and brought it to me.

"I also want to start you on a new AED, although it will most likely not work well, it will help stabilize your seizures for a while. It's called *Beriveracetam*. Going over your list of medications, and knowing their properties very well, the *Lacosamide* has similar AED properties as the *Oxcarbazepine* which could be why it's not working well. So, I want to get you off of that and onto the new medication today." He explained to me the instructions for both of the AEDs, "I don't like to have patients immediately stop their AEDs, I like to have them slowly go down or up in dosage first, so let me explain. I'll print this for you as well:

"New Medication Instructions:

- *Continue current AED Oxcarbazepine 1500mg/1500mg and Zonisamide 400mg daily*

- *First Week – Beriveracetam 100mg tab/2x daily,*

Continue Lacosamide 200mg tab/2x daily

- *Second Week – Beriveracetam 100mg tab/2x daily,*

Decrease Lacosamide to 100mg/2x daily

- *Third week – Beriveracetam 100mg tab/2x daily, Oxcarbazepine 1500mg/2x daily,*

Zonisamide 400mg at bedtime daily, STOP Lacosamide

So, these are the instructions for your new medication dosages. I'll be back to grab the list for you." Doctor Devrat walked out, grabbed the list, and handed it to me.

I stared at the list confused, and really concerned at how many medications I was going to be taking at that time.

"So, I would like to see you back in clinic in two months and we will see where we are then." He said before we all stood up, shook hands, and walked out. My father and I went to pick up the new medication from the pharmacy, as it had been sent in during my appointment, so it was ready for pick up.

By the time we got home, we sat down with my mother and we explained everything to her. The change in AEDs, again, my new diagnosis of Intractable Epilepsy, and the possibility of brain surgery and going through the invasive testing and candidacy for surgery.

HOPE WITHIN ME

After we had explained it all to my mother, I went upstairs to my bedroom and shut the door. I wanted to feel fine, like everything was okay, but the truth at the time was I was scared, hurt, and lost. I threw the papers Doctor Devrat had given me on my bed and I fell to my knees and cried. I cried for myself and for everything I had been through for half of my life. I let my heart and soul cry for everything. I longed for an answer, for something, for hope. I cried for God to show up, I longed for it. I needed and wanted Him to do something in me that I wasn't able to do. I knew I needed to trust in something and put my Faith somewhere, and I gave it all up, all to God. I knew if there was something, someone who could do anything it was Him. That afternoon I cried more than I had ever cried in my entire life. I felt like I had been told I would die soon. Having been told I had Intractable Epilepsy, where no matter what they did, how many AEDs I was given, it was never going to work. I needed an answer, a light, I needed hope.

TESTING BEGINS - 2020

It was January of 2020 by the time I was able to schedule my first appointment with the *Medical·*

Center for diagnostic testing to see if I would be a good candidate for Epilepsy surgery. I was

nervous, anxious, broken, and scared. I was hoping I would be a candidate, but I knew the

process and road ahead to that answer was a long one, so I knew I needed to be patient as it

required me to wait. The first test Doctor Devrat had ordered was an outpatient EEG

(electroencephalogram). I had only had one EEG before, which was back in high school, but it

was a Video EEG where I needed to be hospitalized for a week. So, I had never had an outpatient

one before where I was to go just for a couple of hours and then leave. It was scheduled for

Wednesday, January 22. I went alone that time, as both of my parents worked during the week. I

ended up taking a ridesharing service, which I was used to as I always did for getting places when my parents weren't able to take me around.

The appointment started at one o'clock in the afternoon that Wednesday. It wasn't in the main hospital, but instead at a diagnostic lab about a mile away. I checked in half an hour early for my appointment at the front desk. It was odd, as I was the only patient there, but I waited what seemed like an hour. I then heard a women's voice call my name.

"James?"

I stood up and proceeded to walk to the door. I smiled at her.

"Can I get your date of birth?" She asked before I walked in.

"June 1."

"Come on in. We are going to the room to your left."

"Okay." I looked back at her to make sure.

She gestured, "Yeah, that one."

It was a room two times as big as my own bedroom, with a recliner in the center of the room. There were also monitors to the right of the recliner that I assumed were for monitoring the EEG. I walked into the room farther, then I heard the room door shut.

"Alright James, you can have a seat in the recliner there, and make yourself comfortable. Have you ever done an EEG before?"

"Yes, but only a Video EEG about seven or eight years ago." I said as I sat down in the oversized recliner.

"Okay, then this is nothing new. This will work the same, but it will only last a couple of hours. Our goal today is to get you to have a seizure during your time here."

"Okay." I said nervously.

Once I was comfortable, she pulled out a small box with wires and started to apply them to different areas of my head. As she did, I noticed different lines start to appear on the monitor, which I only assumed was my brain's electrical activity. After she finished applying all of the wires, she wrapped my head with a gauze type of wrapping to keep them from moving. It reminded me of the Video EEG I did back in high school. She then handed me a button.

"Okay James, do you remember what this button is for?"

"If I feel anything, or like I'm having or about to have a seizure I should push it?" I half asked and told her.

"Correct, that way it will mark it in those lines there on the monitor screens." She pointed to them and confirmed with me.

"Now, I want to start by having you sleep for about fifteen to twenty minutes. I want your brain to relax and calm down so we can see what it is doing during that time. So, go ahead and try to relax and sleep." She said with a calming voice. She dimmed the lights and had me close my eyes.

What I assumed was fifteen or twenty minutes later, the lights faded back to normal which woke me up.

JAMES VALENCIA

"Alright James, how do you feel now?"

"I feel good." I said as I tried to adjust to the brightness of the room again.

"That was about twenty minutes and I don't see any seizure activity yet. The next thing we are going to do are flashing lights." She pulled out a stand with a light on it, then put a pair of glasses on her head. "We are going to do two or three sessions of these, each one lasting one minute. Are you ready?"

"Yeah, I'm ready."

"Okay, let's begin." She turned the light on. She watched the monitor carefully for any electrical activity and I stared directly at the light. It began to flash in slow strobes at first. Then it grew a little faster. During the session, it reminded me of all the times I went to clubs with friends from college, which was odd that I was thinking of that at the time. Then suddenly, the strobes became extremely fast and the lights started to bother my eyes.

"Should my eyes be closed or open?" I finally asked.

She looked at me, and noticed my eyes were open. She immediately turned the light off. "Yes. During these sessions, your eyes should be closed the entire time. I didn't even realize they were open. I should have made that clear at the beginning."

Once my eyes were closed, and she saw them closed, she started the session again. The strobes began slow again then became faster as time went on. We did three sessions of them. But at the end, there was still no seizure activity.

"Okay James, I want you to close your eyes again and try to relax and sleep for about five minutes. That way your brain can calm down from all of the activity it just encountered with the lights." She had me rest before we moved to the next test. "Okay James, how do you feel now?"

"I feel good." I replied.

"You don't feel like you had a seizure while resting?"

"I don't think so."

"Okay. Well, the next thing we are going to do is hyperventilation. We will do just two sessions of this, each one being one minute each. What this test does is slow the brain rhythm down and can trigger a seizure. So, let's see if this works for you. First, I want you start by taking deep breathes then start to get faster mid-way through. I will let you know when to speed up and slow down your hyperventilating."

"Okay." I remembered hating this test from the Video EEG back when I was in high school, but I knew if I wanted the surgery I needed it to work that time. As we went through both sessions, again, no seizure activity. Everything was normal.

"Okay, great job on the hyperventilating! I didn't see anything out of the ordinary, but I will look over all of the EEG tests and the time you were here today and send the results to Doctor Devrat so he can also go over them too. You are all done for the day James, good job today." She started to take off each wire from my head and clean the glue she used for them from my hair. She walked me out of the room, and I was on my way home.

JAMES VALENCIA

. . . . .

I had officially started *Master Chorale Singers* again by the end of January and early

February. It felt good singing in choir again, especially after all of the news I had received in the

November and December. Rehearsals were all I looked forward to at that point. That was all I

had, rehearsals and doctor's appointments. We had been working diligently on hard music that

spring, and the concert approached that March. However, little did we know a global pandemic

was headed our way. A global virus had spread throughout countries beyond anyone's wildest

dreams and people were getting sick. By March of 2020, our spring concert was cancelled due to

the pandemic, which made me sad and more broken. But I didn't let that stop me from holding

onto the faith and hope I still had. I knew I just needed to focus on my surgery.

It was time for my follow-up appointment with Doctor Devrat on Thursday, March 19.

However, due to the pandemic, my appointment had turned into a video conference with him

instead of a face to face, as the virus was a respiratory virus that was spreading around the globe.

So, I logged into my computer that Thursday morning and we met. The first thing we did was go

over the Outpatient EEG tests I did on January 22.

"Hello James. So, your EEG results came back normal."

"Oh, okay." Part of me happy but disappointed as well. "So where do we go from here?"

"I want to do more diagnostic testing. So, I want to admit you into the EMU (Epilepsy

Monitoring Unit) at the *Medical Center* for about six or seven days and have you do a Video

EEG with us."

"Will this be more beneficial than the outpatient EEG?"

"So, what the Inpatient Video EEG at the EMU will do is help better characterize and

localize the events and seizures you are having. I also want to explain that during your admission

there, medications will be tapered off, you will be sleep deprived, and you will undergo other

induction procedures including hyperventilation, photic stimulation, exercise, and more in order

to induce seizures. This will help me and the panel at the *Medical Center* gain additional

information about the precise nature and localization of your events and seizures you are having.

Your stay may be shorter or longer depending on when you have a seizure, and we get what we

are looking for." Doctor Devrat explained all of this to me.

"Okay." All of that information both excited and made me nervous at the same time.

"How are your seizures going right now?"

"I am still having them every week. If I'm lucky, every other week."

"Okay, so let's raise your *Zonisamide* 100mg at night starting tonight then. So, continue

taking everything else as normal, *Oxcarbazepine 1500mg 2x/daily, Lacosamide 100mg 2x/daily,*

Beriveracetam 100mg 2x/daily. Now, starting tonight, instead of *400mg* take *500mg* of

Zonisamide. So, instead of four capsules, take five capsules tonight."

"Okay, that sounds good." I said.

JAMES VALENCIA

"Okay James, I sent the referral over to the *Medical Center*, and to you as well. Wait a few days before calling to make the appointment. I will see you in a couple of months then, if not sooner at the *Medical Center* in the EMU." We said our good-byes before we ended our calls on our computers.

I was hopeful for the Video EEG I was going to schedule. All I had to do was wait before I called the hospital to make the appointment. As I waited, I prayed. I longed for a miracle. In the back of my head, I reminded myself to be patient through the process and testing I was headed through. I knew it was going to be a long road and journey ahead me. But I kept my head held high as I looked for a light somewhere through the darkness I had been in for many years. I held onto the tiny sliver of hope I had left within me.

SCHEDULING ISSUES - SPRING 2020

It had been a few days after the appointment with Doctor Devrat when I tried to schedule the Inpatient Video EEG. However, due to the global pandemic, medical centers across the state and country were being closed down with limited allowance of admittance. Every few days during March and April I called the *Medical Center* EMU and tried to schedule the test, but it kept being delayed by weeks. They didn't know when they were going to re-open the *Medical Center*. I was frustrated, not knowing when I was going to be able to schedule the test, as the referral was only good for six months before it needed to be cleared by Doctor Devrat and the insurance again. Still, I made sure to call every few days, setting reminders in my phone so I didn't forget.

May arrived, and the pandemic grew worse throughout the world and country. Worried at how long the process was taking just to see if I was a candidate for surgery, I called every day in

May. On May 5, I started by talking with the *Medical Center* EMU appointments person who said she'd call me back. I hung up my phone, not expecting a call back from her. Soon after, my mother came home from work and we talked for a bit, and I told her how the appointments person said she would call me back, but I didn't believe it. But, not even twenty minutes later, my phone rang again.

"Hello?" I asked, not recognizing the number.

"Hi, may I speak to James?"

"This is he."

"Hi, I'm calling from the *Medical Center*. I'm with the EMU appointments, we spoke earlier."

"Oh yes, hi."

"Hi James. So, we actually, if you are able to and want, can have you come in starting tonight. I know that is last minute, but we have a free bed available. Or you can come in tomorrow morning if that is better?"

"Um, I need to talk to my mother first if you don't mind."

"No problem. Just give me a call back no later than four o'clock this evening."

"Okay. I'll call you right back. Thank you." I hung up the phone.

I had to explain to my mother what I had just been told and offered. I knew I needed to take it. Not many people were allowed into the *Medical Center* during the pandemic, so it was a a blessing in disguise. I knew she would be sad though, especially as no guests or family members would even be allowed to walk me into the building.

"Who was that?" She asked.

"It was the appointments person. She found a day for me to do my Inpatient Video EEG."

"That's good! What day is it, and what time?"

I gulped, I knew it was last minute for her, and it was going to make her sad. "She said I can be admitted tonight."

"Tonight? Your dad isn't even home from work yet."

"I know, but I need to call her back and let her know. She hasn't given me details yet. She also said tomorrow morning. That might work too. I might just tell her I want that. I'll be there for six to seven days." my mother's eyes started to water.

"Yeah, if you can try to ask for tomorrow morning, that would be better." She choked on her words.

"Okay, I'm going to call her back right now then to make sure I get that day." I went to call the appointments person back.

"Hi, this is James Valencia."

"Hi James."

"Hi, is it still okay if I be admitted tomorrow morning?"

"Yes it is. There will be a few things you need to do before coming in though."

"Okay, let me grab a pen and paper. I'm ready."

"Okay, your admittance tomorrow will be Wednesday May 6 – 11. At 9:30am you will go across the street from the *Medical Center* to get tested for the virus before entering the hospital. After you are tested, wait about an hour in the parking lot, and we will call you about the results of the virus test. If it's negative, you will be allowed into the *Medical Center*."

"Okay, where do I go from there once I'm in the *Medical Center*?"

"When you get to the front door, only you will be allowed into the building, no one else. Not even parents. They will screen your temperature and ask for your name. Tell them you are being admitted into the EMU. Then, just go to the elevators and go to floor nine. That is the adult neurology floor."

"Okay, so at 9:30am get tested for the virus, wait an hour. You will call me and verify my results. If cleared I can go to the *Medical Center*. Then, I go to the front door, where only I'm allowed in, they will screen my temperature. I will let them know I am going to EMU, and going to floor nine, adult neurology. Correct?" I asked and confirmed.

"Correct James. That's all the instructions I have for you. We will see you tomorrow, May 6, at the *Medical Center* EMU."

"Okay, thank you so much. Bye." I hung up my phone. I looked at my mother who I noticed was crying as she heard my part of the conversation.

"So, what time do we take you tomorrow?" my mother asked. I sat next to her.

"There's a few things I need to do first before being admitted." I showed her the list and explained what the process looked like due to the pandemic.

"So, I can't even go in with you? Not even to check you in?"

"No. Only patients, and we can't have visitors either."

"I texted my supervisor from work to let her know I can't come in tomorrow that way I can take you. So, we can leave the house at 9:00am? That way we can get to the virus testing site by the correct time?"

"Yeah, that sounds good."

My dad arrived home later that evening, and we both went over what had been scheduled, and explained what the process of admittance was going to look like. He seemed okay with it; he knew it had to be done. I was able to tell they were both sad I'd be gone and not able to see me for almost a week though. I hugged my dad and said bye, as he left for work early in the mornings, and went upstairs that night. I packed loose and comfortable clothes to take with me to the EMU. I went to bed that night, excited, nervous, and waited for the next day to arrive.

VIDEO ELECTROENCEPHALOGRAM - MAY 6, 2020

It was the morning and day of my Video EEG. My mother and I were downstairs in our living room as we were getting ready to leave and head to the virus testing site. It took us probably twenty minutes to get to the testing site, so we arrived early. But it was fine because there was a line to get tested. I needed to stay in the car while I got tested, so I rolled the car window down and the person asked for my name. Once I confirmed my name, they took a long swab and put it up my nose as far as they could. Then, they took another one and swabbed my throat. It was super uncomfortable. Once it was done, my mother and I drove across the street to the *Medical Center* parking lot and waited for the EMU call. It would be an hour, so we sat and listened to music.

"Since we have an hour, let's go get something to drink." My mother said.

"Okay. Yeah, because it will be a while before they call me."

We drove to the nearest fast-food place where we both bought unsweetened iced teas. We sat in their parking lot and listened to music on low volume.

"Do you have everything you need? Clothes, medication, toothbrush?" My mom asked.

"Yeah I do. And I think they're giving me medication; I don't think I use my own. But I brought mine in the original bottles just in case."

It was ten minutes later, my phone started to ring. "Wow, that's early."

"Is that them?"

"I don't know. I'm going to answer it."

"Okay."

"Hello?" I answered.

"Hi, may I speak to James?"

"This is he."

"Hi James, I just wanted to let you know your results came back negative. So, you are able to check into the *Medical Center* now until noon."

"Okay, great. Thank you!"

"Okay, see you soon. Bye."

I hung up the call and told my mother. "They said I can check in now. That was fast."

"Okay then, are you ready?"

"Yeah." I said. So, we headed to the *Medical Center*. As we drove up to the front door, I grabbed my bag from the back seat and put a face mask on, as it was required due to the pandemic. I hugged my mother before I left the car.

"I love you son."

"I love you too." I said as I waived to her before I shut the car door.

I walked to the front door where I was stopped by two men with touchless temperature readers. They screened my temperature and asked why I was there.

"I'm being admitted to the EMU in adult neurology on the ninth floor." I said before they let me into the building. I proceeded to the elevators and made my way up to EMU where I checked in and the day nurse showed me to the room I was going to be staying in for the rest of the week.

"Okay James, this will be the room you will be staying in. Room one." He said. "And this will be your bed right here. I'll give you some privacy for a couple minutes but go ahead and change into this gown right here and we will get you set up for the Video EEG."

"Okay. Thank you." I changed into the gown and put my normal clothes into my bag.

"Alright James, are you ready?" The nurse asked before coming in.

"Yeah."

"Okay, cool. Go ahead and get comfortable on the bed. I'll get you some more pillows. Do you know how to work the television?"

"Yeah I do."

"Okay, awesome. So, how long have you had seizures?"

"It will be ten years in about a month."

"Oh wow. Well, hopefully this Video EEG helps you out man. You're young. You go to school or work?

"I finished my Bachelor's and Master's already. And I taught choir for a while, but I had to stop because I was having seizures."

"Wow, a Master's at twenty-three? Impressive. I'm twenty-seven and thinking of going back to school myself. Well, we're going to do everything we can to help you out and make you have a seizure while you're here." We both laughed, "probably the only time having a seizure is a good thing. The technician should be here soon to attach the wires and set up the monitors. I'll see you in a bit bud."

"Okay, thanks." I said, as he left the room.

Something about his demeanor and the way he genuinely talked calmed me, made me confident that they would be able to help. Not long after the day nurse left, the EEG technician came into the room to attach the wires and electrodes to my head and set everything up. She placed the electrodes on different parts of my scalp. I watched the monitor, the way I did in January with the Outpatient EEG, and saw the lines start appearing one by one. After everything was placed, she took as much gauze as she could and wrapped my head with it so none of the electrodes and wires were exposed and were able to move. She then handed me the button, which I was to use anytime I felt like I was about to have or had a seizure. I remembered that from January and back during the high school Video EEG. She left the room once everything was set up and I was comfortable and had everything I needed for the week.

The day nurse came back into the room after she left.

"Hey James, how are you doing? It looks good on you. You look like a mummy with all that gauze wrapped around your head though." We laughed. "Did she give you a button and explain how to use it?"

"Yeah, she did."

"Cool. Doctor Devrat should be here soon to explain how he wants to do things during your observation throughout the week. So, for now just relax and he'll be here shortly."

"Okay." I pulled out my laptop, as I had brought it to stream movies and television shows instead of watching hospital television. Plus, I had been in the middle of a television series.

Later that evening, I heard a knock on the door. Doctor Devrat walked into the room.

"Good evening James. How are you doing?" He asked as he looked around at me.

"I'm doing good." I closed my laptop and set it aside.

"Alright, it looks good. Everything is set up. So, I wanted to go over how this week will go with you."

"Okay."

"You are scheduled to be here for six days, but it may or may not be shorter or longer depending on if and when we can get you to have a seizure. Our goal is to get you to have at least two or three seizures total. Also, I want to explain what I plan to do while you are here. Today, the first day, I want to start by sleep depriving you. So, the nurses will make sure you don't sleep until around one or two o'clock in the morning. Then, tomorrow on the second day, I will sleep deprive you again, and push it until three o'clock in the morning. I will also add flashing lights and hyperventilation. That's all I have planned right now, so we will go from there."

"Okay." I nodded.

"I will be back every so often to check in on you and keep you updated. Bye-bye James."

"Bye." I said.

I was nervous. Just the thought of a seizure made me nervous, but I knew that was the reason I was there. It was the ultimate goal of finding the solution. By the time my normal bedtime came, which was around eight o'clock in the evening, I started to get tired. The nurses kept me awake though. I watched movies which helped pass the time. Finally, the night nurse came in and told me it was okay to sleep. I fell asleep, what seemed, instantly. But before I knew it, I was woken up by the day nurse. It was a different day nurse this time.

"Good morning James. I'm sorry to wake you up."

"It's okay."

"Here's your medication for the morning." She handed me a cup full of pills. "So, it says here we will be doing more sleep depriving tonight, flashing lights, and hyperventilation."

"Okay." I said before I swallowed the pills.

It was around two o'clock in the afternoon when someone walked in with a light on wheels. All I remember thinking to myself was, *make sure to keep my eyes closed.*

"Hello James."

"Hi."

"We are going to do some more testing. Are you ready?"

"Yeah, I'm ready." I adjusted the hospital bed.

"Okay, we are going to do three sessions of these, each one minute long. Make sure your eyes are closed while doing this."

At least this person told me to close my eyes this time, was all I thought before the lights started. We did three sessions. Each one bothered my eyes, but I felt nothing afterwards.

"How do you feel now James?"

"I feel fine."

"You don't feel like you had a seizure or any different? If not that's totally fine."

"No, it just bothered my eyes."

"Okay. I'm going to take this light out, then I'll be back to do another test with you. We are going to do hyperventilating next. I'll be back, but for now hold onto the button just in case and rest your eyes."

"Okay." I watched her wheel the light out of the room before I shut my eyes. I heard a knock on the door again.

"James, are you ready?"

I opened my eyes. "Yeah, I'm ready."

"Okay, so we are going to be doing hyperventilation for three sessions, each one minute long. You will start slow, then grow faster. I will tell when to go faster and slower."

We did three sessions of hyperventilation. This test was tricky for me, as my mouth was constantly getting dry, but I got through it.

"Good job James. We are all done for today."

"Okay, thanks." I said.

Not even a minute after she left the room though, I felt the feeling. The rising sensation in my mid body and chest. I grabbed the button and pushed it. Before I knew it, I was surrounded by nurses who were talking to each other as I came out of my seizure.

"James, are you okay?" One of the nurses asked.

"Yeah, I think."

"Do you know you just had two seizures right now?"

"I think I do. I remember trying to grab the button, but I don't remember if I pushed it."

"You did push it. Good job."

"Oh, okay."

"Do you know where you are and what day it is?"

"The *Medical Center* and May 7."

"And do you know why you're here?"

"To do a Video EEG."

"Good."

The nurses started to talk to each other.

"What was he doing last?"

"He had just finished his tests. He finished hyperventilation last, but not even a few minutes ago."

"Put that into his notes, and we'll contact Doctor Devrat."

"Hey, James. We're going to get you some water, okay? And dinner will be here shortly."

"Okay."

I slept for a few hours after the nurses left the room. Before I knew it, dinner had arrived, and it was time to eat. I had been hungry and exhausted from the seizures. I ate *everything* they had given me that evening for dinner. I pulled out my laptop again to watch a few television shows to take my mind off of my seizures, as it had made me depressed for a bit. However, it wasn't long before I heard a knock on the door again. I looked over and it was Doctor Devrat. He walked into the room. I set my laptop down to the side of the bed.

"Hello James. How are you feeling today?"

"I'm feeling fine. Tired."

"Yes, I heard you had two seizures today, impressive. I looked at it and it was blurry as to where it was coming from. It looked like one of the temporal lobes but wasn't too clear. But, we still have time, especially since it's day two. So, since you had one right after the flashing lights and hyperventilating, I want to keep that for day three as well. So here is the plan for tonight, and tomorrow. Tonight, instead of keeping you up until three o'clock, let's make it one o'clock again since you had a seizure today. I also want to stop your *Zonisamide* and *Brivaracetam* completely tonight. Then Starting in the morning, no medication at all. Completely off."

"So, nothing at all by tomorrow morning?" I asked nervously.

"Yes, I'm stopping the last two medications that were recently added first. Then stopping the older medications next."

"Okay." I gulped.

"Tomorrow, day three, you'll be tapered off medications, you'll do flashing lights and hyperventilation, and we'll probably add sleep deprivation depending on how things go. That's the plan. For now, relax and if you need anything the nurses are all here to help. Bye-bye James." Doctor Devrat walked out of the room. All I heard was his footsteps and beeps of machines.

HOPE WITHIN ME

That night was just as long as the previous night.. It was hard to stay awake, especially after I had just had a seizure earlier. I waited until the nurses told me I was allowed to go to sleep though. It felt good to fall asleep. The only good part about being able to sleep that night was that no one needed to wake me up early the next day for medication, as I would be completely tapered off of it. I spent most of the following day with the button on my side, nervous. But I also enjoyed the day by watching movies and television shows to fill the sadness and loneliness I felt being there in the *Medical Center*.

Once again, I heard a knock on the door. It was two o'clock again. It was time to start the tests. It was the same person as the previous day.

"Hi James, how are you doing today?" she asked.

"I'm doing good."

"Good. We are going to do the same thing as yesterday, okay? Three sessions of flashing lights and three sessions of hyperventilating. Each will be one minute. We will start with flashing lights again."

"Okay." We proceeded through the three sessions before we moved to hyperventilating.

"Okay, remember, start slow then get faster. I will let you know when to go faster and slower." We went through all three sessions of hyperventilating before we finished.

The person wheeled the light out again and left the room. I pulled out my laptop to watch more television series. I made sure to hold the button close just in case I felt anything. Before I was able to login to my laptop, there it was again. The rising sensation. I hated it. I pushed the button. I heard nurses out in the nurse area outside of the room call out to each other for help.

"James Valencia is having a seizure."

They came into the room to help.

"James are you okay?"

"Yeah, I'm fine." My seizure started to end.

"Do you know where you are and what day it is?" A nurse asked. But there it was, the feeling again. It came fast though, no aura or warning sign, it just happened.

"James are you okay?" a nurse kept asking.

"He's not responding. That's his second seizure." I vaguely remember her saying to another nurse while I started to come out of the second seizure. But again, I felt another feeling, that time there was an aura.

All I heard before the next seizure, "Room one, bed one is having a seizure again!"

I woke up surrounded by multiple nurses. I looked around the room confused, tired, and not knowing what had happened.

"James are you feeling better now?" a male nurse asked me.

"Yeah? I'm just really tired and confused."

"You had three seizures back-to-back. So, what we did to help you was give you some liquid AED medication through your intravenous line because you were going into what appeared to be Non-Convulsive Status Epilepticus. We wanted to make sure you didn't go into Convulsive Status Epilepticus by preventing a Tonic-Clonic seizure, so giving this medication was our only option and was the safest thing for you."

"Okay."

"So, go ahead and keep sleeping if you want. Dinner will be here shortly."

I fell asleep for a while until dinner arrived. I wasn't too hungry, as I was more tired that evening than anything, So, I waited to eat. But not long after eating dinner, I heard a knock on the door.

"Hello James. I heard you had quite a day." Doctor Devrat walked into the room.

"Yeah."

"Three seizures in one day. Well, I have some good news about all of those seizures."

"You do?"

"All three of the seizures that occurred today were crystal clear. They showed up in the exact same spot on the EEG. They were all happening within the right temporal lobe. That's a good thing for you, and I'll tell you why. If someone has multiple seizures that occur in different places in the brain, then there's no focus of those seizures, they're just random and will be hard to remove. For you though, because they're all happening in the right temporal lobe in that one area, that means there is something there that is causing it and can most likely be removed. Even your first seizure, yesterday, came from the same area, it was just blurry. Today, crystal clear."

"Okay, so it's all in the right temporal lobe."

"Correct. So, I will make a report to bring to the panel here at the *Medical Center*. I want to start you back on your normal AEDs tonight. I think we can get ready to discharge you either tonight or tomorrow morning. The next thing I want to do with you is get a PET Scan."

"What's a PET Scan? What does that do?"

"A PET Scan uses a radioactive tracer to show anything abnormal in the brain. So, if anything abnormal is going on in the right temporal lobe, it will make the scan glow up immediately and reveal what is going on. That's the next test I want from you. For now, I want you to rest, we'll get you back on your medications, and get you home soon. This was a remarkably successful Video EEG James. Bye-bye."

"Bye Doctor Devrat" I said before he walked out.

I was proud of how well it had gone, especially compared to the Video EEG back when I was in high school. And the thought of being able to go home the following morning made me happy, so I pulled out my laptop to watch more movies. But not even an hour later there it was, the feeling again. The rising sensation in my upper chest. This seizure was different though. Because Doctor Devrat had told me about the possibility of going home that day, I had been excited to go home. With the button in my hand still, I stood up from the bed itself when a nurse noticed. She came to help me sit back down on the bed. I had thought I was able to just walk right out of the room to leave. But by standing up, I had ripped out some of the electrodes from

214

my hair. By the time I had come out of the seizure, I realized some of the leads on my head were missing. So, the EEG technician came to replace them. I apologized for messing it up, but she was nice about it.

I was discharged from the *Medical Center* the following morning. I was given instructions on my medications, a referral to get a PET Scan, and also information on Convulsive and Non-Convulsive Status Epilepticus. I met my father that time at the front door. I was wheeled out in a wheelchair. When I arrived home from the *Medical Center* that morning, I sat down with my parents and told them everything. They were shocked at how many seizures I had during my stay, but glad everything had gone well according to Doctor Devrat.

I was more hopeful than ever, especially with all the seizures I had during my stay. And although I was having just as many seizures on a weekly basis, my hope kept growing stronger every day. I started to feel confident that no matter what happened, or how things worked out, it was going to be okay.

PET SCAN - FRIDAY MAY 29, 2020

I had been able to schedule the PET Scan without any trouble in May. The appointment was set

for eleven o'clock in the morning on May 29. I was given two instructions to follow before going

into the diagnostic lab, which was to eat a low carbohydrate and high protein dinner. The high

protein content was to help the radioactive tracer (Fludeoxyglucose F-18) attach itself to it and

help it find any abnormalities hidden in my brain. Also, I wasn't allowed to brush my teeth,

drink, or eat anything the morning of the test, as the fluoride in any toothpaste or mouthwash

would mess with the tracer and food would make the tracer less effective.

It was ten o'clock in the morning when my parents took me to the diagnostic lab to be

tested. They waited in the car as I went in by myself. I was stopped at the door, my temperature

was checked before I was allowed in, and I checked in. I sat down in the waiting area as I patiently waited to be called back. I had researched what the test was before going into the

diagnostic lab, so I knew somewhat of what it was going to look like, but I was still nervous,

especially being alone. Then, twenty minutes later I heard my name called from a door.

"James?"

I looked around the room. Why? I'm not sure, as there was only me. Probably more out

of nervousness.

"James Valencia?"

I proceeded to the door. "Hi" I smiled at the man.

"Date of birth please?"

"June 1."

"Follow me. We are going into this room to the left."

I walked into a small room. There was a bed and a scale. He weighed me first before he

had me put my belongings into a locker and locked them up. Then, I laid down on the bed.

"Okay James, have you had anything to drink, eat, or brushed your teeth this morning?"

"No. I did have a sip of water, but just to take my AEDs. They said it was okay to do that

if it was a tiny bit of water for my medication."

"Yes, that's fine. So, I'm having you lay down to rest your brain. We will do this for

about fifteen minutes before heading over to the PET Scan. I will be putting a warm towelette

over your eyes and blanket over you as well. About five minutes through, I will come back in and inject the tracer into your arm. Try to relax and keep your eyes closed. I'm going to dim the lights now, okay?"

"Okay." I closed my eyes, with the towelette over them, and tried to relax.

I didn't know how much time had passed, as I felt like I had fallen asleep, but I soon heard the room door open. The towelette was still over my eyes.

"James, how are you doing?"

"I'm doing good."

"I'm going to inject the tracer now." I felt him lift up my arm and feeling for a vein. He then injected me with the tracer. "Alright, I'll be back in a bit. Keep the towelette over your eyes." I heard the door shut.

The door opened soon, and the towelette was lifted from my eyes. The brightness of the room had caught me off guard.

"Okay James, we are going to head over to the PET Scan room now." He helped me stand up and off the bed. We headed down the hallway to a giant room with a machine that was typically used for MRIs. It was going to be the same as an MRI, only I had a radioactive tracer inside my body.

"So, James, I'm assuming you've had many MRIs before. This will work the exact same way. You will be in here for probably thirty to forty minutes until we get the pictures we need. Okay?"

He helped me lay down onto the skinny bed that pulled out of the round machine. He put a warm blanket over me to keep me warm. All of the warm blankets and towels were to help the tracer work better. He handed me a pair of ear plugs, which never worked, that I put into my ears. Then, like every MRI I had done before, he put the cage over my face to keep my head from moving. He then handed me a button, in case I needed to get out of the machine, and proceeded to push the bed into the machine. I then heard the noise I had grown fond of, the sound going round and round, the "swishing" sounds of the magnets going around me. I laid there, staring at the white nothingness in front of me as the noise continued. I decided to close my eyes at a point, prayed the test would hurry up, and that they would be able to find whatever they were looking for, whatever *I* wanted them to look for. Finally, the noise stopped. I opened my eyes as the bed started to move and come out of the machine.

"Alright James, we are all done." He took my ear plugs from me. "you can go back to the locker and gather your belongings now. Do you know how to exit?"

"Yeah, I do. Thanks." I left the room to get my belongings before I exited the building to go back to the car where my parents had still been waiting patiently for me. I couldn't wait to go home and brush my teeth and eat, as it was almost one o'clock by the time I was able to.

. . . . .

HOPE WITHIN ME

June 1, 2020 had soon arrived; I had turned twenty-four years old. Not able to do much because of the pandemic that was raging throughout the world and country, my family and I celebrated at home. My parents had ordered food from a restaurant and picked it up and brought it home. It was a more relaxed birthday, no dressing up or going out. I didn't *really* feel any older. All I thought about at the time was surgery, testing and results almost 24/7.

It was the middle of the day, a few days after my twenty-fourth birthday, when I received a notification on my phone from the *Medical Center*. Everything was done through their online system and cellphone application. I was watching television at the time, but I opened the application to see what it was. It was an appointment that had been scheduled which was odd because I hadn't scheduled anything. Not knowing what it was for, I looked at the details. My jaw dropped with excitement as I jumped up from the couch, as I almost dropped my phone. I wanted to cry. It was a consultation appointment with a neurosurgeon, Doctor Boden, at the *Medical Center*.

When my parents came home later that afternoon, I told them about the notification I had received and the consultation with the neurosurgeon. We were all excited, not knowing what to expect would happen next.

NEUROSURGERY CONSULTATION - THURSDAY JUNE 25, 2020

My consultation appointment with Doctor Boden, the neurosurgeon, had arrived. He was the

Director of Neurosurgery at the *Medical Center,* as well as one of the neurosurgeons who

specialized specifically in Epilepsy surgery. I was scheduled to meet with him that morning of

June 25, 2020. Both of my parents unfortunately weren't able to get the day off, so I told them

both not to worry I would take a ridesharing service to the consultation to meet with him,

considering the fact they weren't going to be able to come inside the office due to the pandemic

that raged around the globe and country. I left for the appointment early, both excited and

nervous. Upon my arrival to the neurosurgery clinic, I was given a sterile mask, asked if I had

been in contact with anyone with a pending virus test or tested positive recently, and my

temperature was taken with a touchless temperature reader before I was allowed to check in.

JAMES VALENCIA

Once I had checked into the office, I sat down in the waiting area. I waited forty minutes, anxious for the news I was going to receive, whether good or bad. The door to the back rooms opened and a nurse called my name. I walked over, confirmed my date of birth and name, and she led me to a small room where I waited again.

I looked around the room I sat in. There were posters of the brain on the wall. I stood up and walked over to the one where it showed the different lobes of the brain. *So, that's the right temporal lobe.* I thought to myself. *That's where Doctor Devrat said my seizures are occurring.* I then heard a knock on the door, so I quickly sat down in the chair again.

"Hello James" a man, probably in his late forties, early fifties said.

"Hello."

"I'm Doctor Boden. I'm the Director of Neurosurgery here at the *Medical Center*, as well as one of the Epilepsy neurosurgeons. I want to go over some of the results and findings of the tests Doctor Devrat, myself, and the panel found."

"Okay." I was scared and nervous.

"I want to start by going over your last MRI. When I went over it, it showed a right temporal anterior encephalocele about **3mm**. Encephaloceles don't occur in many people with Epilepsy but can cause seizures for an exceedingly small number of people with seizures."

"So, what does that mean?"

"I'll explain, but let's move to your Video EEG next."

224

"Okay."

"I promise I'm not ignoring your question; it's all connected. So, with your Video EEG, we identified six seizures all with onset right temporal lobe, again where your encephalocele was found. And finally, your PET Scan, which was extraordinarily clear, identified hypermetabolism in the right anterior temporal lobe."

"Okay." I tried to understand, but knew he was going to explain.

"So, what this means is that there is something there in the anterior part of your right temporal lobe causing you to have seizures, and the increased amount you've been experiencing. And from what we've all agreed and found was that the encephalocele was the root of that. It has been known in some cases that encephaloceles cause Epilepsy and seizures. And in your case, we believe this is what is happening. It couldn't be clearer to the panel."

"So, the encephalocele is the problem?"

"We aren't positive why your seizures started. But we are confident the encephalocele is where your seizures are occurring, and as time progressed, the seizures started to occur more often because of the scar tissue over the encephalocele. What happens when someone has a seizure is that when it is finished, it leaves scar tissue on that part of the brain where it happens."

"Oh, okay." I tried to soak in as much information as I could.

"That is what has happened to you. Your seizures have been happening for so long in that part of your brain that there is so much scar tissue over the encephalocele that the encephalocele has become so irritated it is causing the rise in your frequency in seizures. Also, James, after reviewing all of the information, tests, and the increased frequency of your seizures, the panel is concerned that if left untreated and not well controlled it will put you at an elevated risk of serious injury..." he paused, " ...or eventually even death. Also known as SUDEP, Sudden Unexpected Death in Epilepsy"

With all of the information I had just been given, I was overwhelmed by everything. I didn't know what to think.

"So, what happens next then?" I asked Doctor Boden.

"We are almost certain that by removing that encephalocele, it will correct everything and guarantee you are seizure free and able to live out a normal life."

My heart started to pound a little faster, I had never heard those words in my entire life from a doctor. "Okay."

"So, my question to you, James, is how bad and soon do you want this operation."

"I want it as soon as I can have it. I've lived with this for ten years this coming month now, and I'm tired of it." I said as I tried to hold back emotions.

"Let's do it in a couple of weeks then. I want you to get better. I will have my appointments person come in and make the appointment with you before you leave. But, before that, do you have any questions for me?"

I pulled out my phone to get my list of questions. I had made a list before going into the neurosurgery clinic. "Yes, I have a few questions I wanted to ask you: Like, what kind of surgery will it be? I know there are different kinds."

"For you, it will be a craniotomy of your right temporal lobe. Also known as an Epilepsy resection."

"Okay. And also, how many Epilepsy surgeries do you and the *Medical Center* perform each year, and what is your personal experience?"

"The *Medical Center* performs Epilepsy surgeries multiple times a year. And for myself, I do maybe two or three of these surgeries a week."

"Oh wow. I was thinking maybe two or three a year."

"No, they're quite often here at the *Medical Center*."

"Okay, a few more questions, sorry."

"No, ask away James."

"What functions does this part of the brain control? Like important circuits such as speech, vision, learning, reading, and memory? Also, will this part of the brain grow back? Sorry, I don't know if that happens, where the brain grows back?"

"So, the part of the brain we are planning to remove is where memory is stored. But it shouldn't affect that. We are going to expedite a referral to have you get tested by a neuropsychologist before surgery as well as to help us map out your brain. And no, the brain will not grow back."

"Okay. Will there be short term risks to worry about after surgery or during recovery, like stroke, infection, bone reabsorption, meningitis?"

"As with any surgery, there will be risks of infection. But ultimately there shouldn't be a risk of those things. We will give you guidelines on how to thoroughly clean and take care of the incision after the operation."

"How about long-term functional risks to worry about after surgery? Like any learning deficits, vision problems, physical impairments/motor skills?"

"No, that will all be tested before hand with the neuropsychologist. And the area of the brain we will be operating in for you doesn't include motor skills."

"Okay, cool. Just a couple more questions, I promise."

"You're fine, keep going."

"How long will I be in the hospital after surgery? And how long is the recovery time? Like what will it look like for me since it is brain surgery? Will there be physical therapy?"

"Well, after the operation you will be taken to the Intensive Care Unit for two nights, maybe three before being moved to the Epilepsy Monitoring Unit for maybe one night."

"Really? I don't need to stay any longer?"

"No, the healing time is quite fast with this type of surgery. However, we will be monitoring you closely the first couple of nights in the Intensive Care Unit for any drainage of the brain and for infection. As for therapy, you won't need that."

"Okay. Well, that's all of my questions. Sorry there were so many."

"It's a huge operation James, you can ask as many questions as you want and need." Doctor Boden said.

"I'm all out of them now." I laughed.

"Okay. So, I will go send that neuropsychologist referral out right now and have my appointments person come in to schedule the surgery with you."

Doctor Boden left the room and the appointments person walked in next. She asked what day a good day for me was to have the surgery. I told her any day, the sooner the better. She was able to find me an appointment less than three weeks away. She had also scheduled me a PACE (Pre-Anesthesia Consultation) appointment where they would measure how much anesthesia I would need for the surgery. The last thing she did was give me a referral to get an MRI. The MRI was to clear the operation with the *Medical Center* for legal purposes. She gave me a giant folder with all of that information and the operation information with the referrals. It was overwhelming. But she also gave me her business card and told me if I needed anything to call the office and ask for her since she was Doctor Boden's personal appointments person. She walked out before Doctor Boden returned.

"Alright James, were you able to find a date for surgery?" He asked me.

"Yes." I said. He saw my folder which meant I was set for surgery.

"Let's see what day you have." He scrolled through the computer. "Oh good, a little over two weeks away. July fourteenth. I see your PACE appointment is scheduled already, good. Make sure to get the neuropsychologist, and MRI appointments scheduled and done at least a week before surgery if you can."

"Okay, I will."

"Alright James. I will see you on July fourteenth in the operating room." We stood up, and he walked me out of the room.

I was in awe on my way home that day. When I arrived home, I waited for my parents to get there. And when they did, I told them everything. They were shocked the way I had been. They couldn't believe how soon the operation was going to take place. Something we all thought would take so much longer, had finally become a reality.

I was only weeks away from having Epilepsy surgery. It had all happened so fast. I also knew the most likely cause of my seizures now, after ten years of living with them. Having lived in so much shame, fear, and pain. All of the tears that were shed, I was given a partial answer. I was thankful. All I had to do was get through the surgery and believe it was going to fix everything. The amount of hope and faith I had was strong, but I was also scared at the same time. I knew I had to believe God was going to protect me in whatever happened in the weeks to come. That no matter what happened next, it was the only choice I had left.

Findings from the MRI from October 3, 2019, Video EEG from May 6-9, 2020, and PET Scan from May 29, 2020 reviewed by Doctor Boden and my Epilepsy Panel:

HOPE WITHIN ME

REVIEW OF SYMPTOMS: medically Intractable Onset Impaired Awareness Seizures.

MRI: I reviewed which shows right temporal anterior pole encephalocele.

EMU: identified 6 seizures all with onset right temporal lobe.

FDG-PET Scan: identified clear hypometabolism right anterior temporal lobe.

ASSESSMENT:

Onset Impaired Awareness Seizures, under poor control. Patient was discussed in multidisciplinary Epilepsy conference. He has concordant EEG, MRI, and PET Scan pointing to seizure onset in right anterior temporal lobe related to encephalocele seen in that location.

PLAN:

We discussed risks and benefits of surgery to remove the encephalocele from the right temporal lobe. We discussed that surgery would have an excellent opportunity to completely stop his seizures. He desires to proceed with surgery.

231

PACE - TUESDAY JULY 7, 2020

Twelve days after my neurosurgery consultation, I had my Pre- Anesthesia Consultation (PACE)

appointment. The *Medical Center* had different clinics and offices located in various locations of

the city it was in, so the PACE clinic was located about three miles away from the actual hospital

itself. My parents both worked that day, and it was hard for them to request the day off.

However, my father decided he would take the day off so he could take me to my appointment.

The appointment was in the early afternoon, so we left around eleven o'clock in the morning, so

I was able to go through the procedures set in place upon my arrival to the clinic. They took my

temperature, handed me a sterile face mask, asked questions about who I had been in contact

with before I was cleared to enter the PACE building. Once I had entered the building I checked

in at the door instead of the front desk before being told to sit down in a seat. I waited around ten minutes before I was called to a door across the room.

"James Valencia?" a woman said.

I walked over. "Hi."

"Confirm your date of birth and why you are here please."

"June 1. And a PACE appointment for brain surgery." I was extremely nervous.

"Okay sweetheart, follow me."

I went through the door and to the back where there were offices. She took me to an office where she shut the door once we were inside and had me sit down in a chair across from her. She turned on the computer at the desk she sat at.

"So, James, do you know what this appointment is for?"

"Kind of. Can you explain a little more please?"

"Yes. So, what the anesthesiologist is going to do today is measure how much anesthesia your body can handle during your surgery. It will be so that we keep you safe during the procedure."

"Okay."

"Also, without worrying you too much by saying this, we will be drawing blood from you today. This has been requested by the neurosurgeon and the team that will be working in the operating room. This will be *just in case* if anything goes wrong or you lose too much blood, they have extra blood they will be able to use if you lose too much during the operation."

I couldn't believe what I just heard come out of her mouth. *If anything goes wrong?*

"And James, I want to ask you, have you heard of something called an *Advance Health Care Directive*?"

"No, what is that?"

"An *Advance Health Care Directive* is like a living will or durable power of attorney for healthcare."

I was confused. I had never heard of one before.

"So, James, if something were to happen during the operation, which I'm not saying something will, but if it were and you weren't able to physically communicate and/or make the decision on what to do with your health next, this form would state who would make that decision for you, and what they would do."

"Oh, okay." I had started to get worried at that point. I started to see how real everything had started to become for me.

"It will also give you the power to assign your assets, like money and belongs over to someone if you need to if there were a chance of an accident during the procedure. Which again, there is not a high chance. But it's always good to just have this form in the system for the future. It is completely up to you whether you would like to have it or not. If you would like, I can just print it out, and you can take it home and think about it. And if you want to fill it out, just make sure to bring it to the *Medical Center* the day of your operation."

JAMES VALENCIA

I was overwhelmed and heartbroken with what could happen. But I knew the risks I would be taking if I didn't take the form. "Yes, can I get a copy of the form please."

"Of course, James. Again, we don't believe anything will happen during your operation. We would rather just have it in the system for you, so you are covered and safe if you need it."

"So, I just bring it the day of surgery? And who do I give it too?"

"On the day of surgery, give it to any of the nurses that day and they will take care of it."

"Okay, thank you." She handed me a packet of paper, maybe eight or fifteen pages long I knew I needed to read carefully.

"Okay sweetheart, one of the anesthesiologists will come in now to start talking with you." She walked out of the room.

A man, no older than thirty, walked in next. He sat down at the desk and scrolled through the computer.

"Hi James, how are you doing today?" He asked me.

"I'm doing good." I lied.

"Good to hear. Okay, she went over the form with you. Your medication is listed, that's good." He spoke to himself for a while. "Alright James, so we are going to start by taking you blood pressure, check your oxygen level, take your pulse. Then we will finish by pulling some blood from you." He stood up from the desk. "Okay James, "follow me and we will get started."

"Okay." I grabbed my papers and folder and followed him.

236

HOPE WITHIN ME

We walked out of the office and to a giant room with doctor office beds that were separated by curtains. I sat on a bed while he took my blood pressure, checked my oxygen level, and took my pulse.

"Alright James, I want to give you this packet and another folder." He laughed. "I know you probably have a lot of folders now, but here's another one from PACE. This folder has your Pre-Operation information. Inside it tells you everything you need to know about the day and days before surgery now that you are officially a week away. Including when and where to go."

"Thank you." I looked inside, and there were a lot of papers with times, lists of medications, and foods I needed to stop taking before the operation.

"Okay, I'm going to take you over to the lab area to get your blood work done. You are done with me now." He walked me over to another small room. "I want to wish you luck on your surgery James."

"Thank you."

Once I arrived at the lab area, a lady had me sit down in a chair. She pulled out six tubes she was going to fill with my blood. I was shocked that she filled and took so much. Once the bloodwork was done, I was guided to the exit and left the PACE clinic. I couldn't have been happier. I got back into the car with my dad, as he had waited the entire time. I told him everything that was said. Even he was shocked at the paperwork I was given but understood the reason for it. I was overwhelmed by the appointment that day and wanted to get back home.

JULY 8, 2020

The day after my PACE appointment, I had scheduled two appointments I absolutely needed if I wanted the surgery the following week. I had scheduled my neuropsychology appointment and my MRI appointment. They were going to be back-to-back. It was a busy day as they were both less than fifteen minutes apart. But, both offices knew, so they said they would try to do the best they could to accommodate but made no promises for me.

I started the day early in the morning with my neuropsychology appointment. It was going to take around three hours to test. For that test, they tested the different areas of my brain for cognitive deficiencies, strengths, and to map out everything so the surgeons knew what to be cautious of when they operated on my brain. When I walked into the room to meet the neuropsychologist, he seemed friendly. He told me it may or may not take three hours but to be prepared. The test was laid out in two sections:

PART A:

Immediate Memory

Visuospatial/Constructional

Language

Attention

Delayed Memory

PART B:

List Learning Task

Story Memory

Figure Copy

List Orientation

Line Orientation

Picture Naming

Semantic Fluency

Digit Span

Coding

List Recall

List Recognition

Story Recall

Figure Recall

Anything that had to do with figures, spatial, and drawing were my strongest results. He told me that was a good thing, as all of my motor skills and important things I needed for life seemed to be on my left side of the brain, which they weren't going to be operating on. As a musician it had worried me for a bit, but I was relieved at the same time because my motor skills and important necessities for daily life were on the opposite side of the brain. The test only took me two and a half hours before I was able to leave.

I ran over to the MRI building next where I had to get my last MRI completed for the *Medical Center* so they could clear me for the operation. When I arrived at the building, I checked in, and I was led to a room with the MRI machine. It had become so routine for me, I immediately emptied my pockets and put my belongings in the tiny locker they had. I took the key, gave it to the radiologist, and waited until he told me to lay on the MRI bed. Once I was on the bed, the ear plugs were in my ears, the cage was over my face, and I was given the button. I was then pushed into the machine and waited for the oh so familiar sound that would go around me again, taking pictures of my brain. Again, I stared at the white nothingness of the tube as I laid in there, as the pictures were being taken. Once the sound stopped, I was pulled out of the machine and told "Good Job" before I took my belongings and headed home.

It had been a long and exhausting day. I was excited to just go home and do nothing for a

JAMES VALENCIA

while. Two appointments back-to-back. The first one had been two hours long of just pure testing, and the second had been the normal routine of an MRI.

242

MONDAY JULY 13, 2020

The craniotomy was less than twenty-four hours away. However, I had one last appointment to go to. It was an online appointment with my Epileptologist, Doctor Devrat. He had scheduled it so we could have a visit before the operation.

I logged onto my laptop that morning to start the video call with him. I was eager to see what he had to say about everything that had occurred so fast in the past month and a half.

"Good morning James. How are you doing today?" Doctor Devrat asked.

"I'm good. How are you?"

"I'm good too. Are you ready for the surgery tomorrow?"

"Yeah. It's crazy how fast it all happened."

"Yeah, your case was a very interesting one."

243

"Really? How come?"

"All of your tests came out perfectly clear. What actually determined you as a candidate was your PET Scan. If it weren't for that PET Scan, we wouldn't have found the encephalocele that matched your MRI from October of 2019."

"*Really?*"

"Remember how I said the radioactive fluid would make *any* abnormal thing in your brain glow up on the screen? Well, that's exactly what it did with you. It was actually the radiologists who caught it first before the Panel confirmed it. It was remarkable what they found."

I was shocked after I heard the descriptions of all of the tests they had done. Having heard Doctor Boden's and now Doctor Devrat's version of how I became a candidate and what they had found out about my brain was beyond belief.

"Wow, that's incredible. I'm glad I'm able to have this procedure tomorrow. Especially in the midst of the global pandemic right now."

"Yes, it was very timely that we got you into the operating room as soon as possible. That was the one thing we all agreed on. I actually have a patient who had the surgery about six months ago and she's been seizure free ever since."

"Wow, that's amazing and good to know too. I'm really hoping for good results afterwards."

"From what we all found and discussed; I believe you will have excellent results. If not seizure free at the very least, a major improvement. But I'm confident this will fix a lot of what is happening. Alright James, I want to wish you luck for tomorrow. Get some good rest tonight, and I will see you after the operation!"

"Thank you. Bye Doctor Devrat." I hung up the call and closed my laptop.

. . . . .

That day was filled with emotions from my parents, as well as getting prepared for the arrival at the *Medical Center* for the next day. I washed clothes, packed a bag, and made sure all of the paperwork I had been given was inside of it. I spent most the day downstairs with my family. I eventually called the *Medical Center* to confirm the time I needed to arrive. I needed to be there at five o'clock in the morning.

Later that evening, we bought dinner and ate it together on the couch while we watched a movie. We tried not to think too much about the surgery. Finally, when I was headed to bed, I saw my mother sitting in the corner of the couch, and her eyes filled with water. Tears fell down her face. I walked over to her and sat next to her. We both sat there and prayed. Prayed that no matter what was going to happen the next day, something good was going to happen. We said good night before I went to my bedroom where I doublechecked my bag and made sure I had everything I needed for the morning. I laid in my bed, staring at the ceiling. It was a hard night for me to sleep.

God, if you can hear me, please let tomorrow go smoothly. I'm confident it will, but I'm also nervous. I wasn't nervous until today. Please don't let anything bad happen to me. I just want to know what it's like to not live like this anymore. Please protect me, I'm really scared for tomorrow. What makes it worse is that I have to do it alone.

Amen.

RIGHT TEMPORAL LOBE CRANIOTOMY

W/ EPILEPTOGENIC FOCUS - TUESDAY JULY 14, 2020

The day of my surgery had arrived. I woke up at two o'clock in the morning, nervous about how

the next hours would play out for me. I took a good shower, brushed my teeth, then walked

downstairs with my bag. I turned on the television to watch the news. All that was on the news

that morning was information about the virus and the pandemic and how it raged around the

country and world, so I changed it to a cartoon to make me happier. I was already depressed, and

worried. I tried not to show it as I started to hear footsteps from my parent's bedroom as the floor

creaked, so I didn't want them to see me like that. I then heard someone walk down the staircase,

it was my father.

"Hi son, are you all packed and ready?"

"Yeah, I'm ready." I said as I tried not to cry. My father had already showered and gotten ready. He came over to me and gave me a hug.

"I love you son."

"I love you too." I saw his eyes had started to water. We hugged for a while before he walked over to the coffee machine to make coffee. I sat back down on the couch in the living room to continue watching television.

By three o'clock, I had started to wonder when my mother was going to come downstairs. I wanted to be at the *Medical Center* no later than four-thirty, as my check in time was five o'clock. So, if I wanted to be there at the time I wanted, that meant we needed to leave the house around four o'clock.

My mother came downstairs at about three-thirty that morning. She came and sat next to me on the couch. The first thing she did was give me a giant hug. She just held me as tightly as she could for a while.

"Are you packed and ready for today?" she asked.

"Yeah, I think I am."

"Are you nervous or scared?" her eyes started to water up.

"No, if anything I'm more anxious." I lied. The closer each minute had inched towards the procedure, the more scared I had become.

"I love you son. I love you so much." Tears fell down her face as she pulled me in and embraced me.

"I love you too mom" I tried not to cry.

"Alright, are you ready to go?" she asked as she wiped away tears.

"Yeah."

It was four-fifteen o'clock, but before we left the house my mother had gotten my sisters out of bed and we said goodbye to each other. Afterwards, my parents and myself were headed to the *Medical Center.* We arrived there twenty minutes before five o'clock. I gave each of my parents a hug, put on a clean face mask before I walked myself up to the front door alone. No one but me was allowed up to the door. However, when I tried to enter, I was told I needed to wait until five o'clock, so I sat on a bench outside for a few minutes before I called my parents to let them know I was too early. To my surprise, they had been sitting in the car in the parking lot, so I went and sat with them until five o'clock.

At exactly five o'clock I said goodbye to my parents again before I walked over to the front door. I was stopped and screened by two people.

"Are you checking in or visitor?"

"I'm being admitted for inpatient surgery today at five o' clock."

"Okay, step forward please." They took my temperature with the touchless temperature reader. "You're good. Do you know where to go?"

"Not really."

"Do you see that desk right there?" they pointed. "They will lead you."

"Thank you." I walked into the building and to the desk. "Hi, I'm here for inpatient surgery."

"Good morning, what is your name?" a man asked.

"James Valencia."

"Yes, follow me and I will lead you to the check in desk."

I followed him to the check in desk. I was the first patient in line, and soon the line started to grow longer as more people were having surgery, both inpatient and outpatient. I was soon called up to the front desk after they had their system warmed up and ready to go.

"Next?"

I walked up. "Hi, good morning."

"Good morning sweetheart." A woman said. "Can you confirm your name, date of birth and how old you are for me?"

"Yes, James Valencia, June 1 and I'm twenty-four years old."

"Okay, and you are here for an inpatient craniotomy, correct?"

"Yes."

"Now, because the *Medical Center* is not able to have any relatives or visitors inside the hospital due to the virus and pandemic going on, we have nurses and a text message system set in place. This alerts family members when surgery begins, how the process is going throughout the surgery, and when you are in recovery. This is for the ease of mind for your family. Do you want or have anyone who you want to include in this?"

"Yes, can I have my mother included with that please?"

"Yes sweetheart. Is the emergency number we have on file for her correct?" She read

back the number.

"Yes it is."

"Okay, so throughout the process and day, she will be getting updates, including when

you have checked in which is right now."

"Okay, thank you so much."

"Okay sweetheart, go ahead and take a seat, and someone will come back to get you."

I walked over to a seat and sat down. I watched as multiple people checked in that

morning. I wondered what each person was going to have a procedure on. The only person I

came to find out was a lady who sat across from me and started to talk to me. We shared about

our stories and what we were there for. She was there for heart surgery. As we sat there, we

prayed together. We prayed God would be there for each of us as we went through two major

surgeries that morning.

I waited thirty minutes after I had checked in before someone came out to the waiting

area and brought me back to the Pre-Operation area.

"James? James Valencia?"

I stood up and walked over to the nurse. "Good morning."

"Follow me."

I followed her. We walked to an elevator where we went up to the Pre-Operation room. Once I was in the room, I was given a gown, hospital socks, and sticky pads for my buttocks as I was going to be on the operation table for at least four hours. I took off all of my clothes and changed into the gown, put on the socks, and the nurse put the sticky pads on my buttocks. I then remembered about the *Advance Health Care Directive*. I pulled the form out of my bag and waited for the nurse to come back from her computer in the corner.

"Excuse me, I have a form for you. I was told to give you this from the PACE clinic."

She took the form. "Oh yes, thank you. I will scan this into the system right now and give this back. Give me a few minutes."

"Okay." I waited probably ten minutes before she came back.

"Okay, it is scanned into the system now. I'm just going to stick the form into your bag. Is that okay?" She put the form in my bag for me, as my bed had been lifted and the bag was on the floor. "Also, I put a tag around your bag, so the nurses know to take your bag to the *Intensive Care Unit*. I want your bag to follow you after surgery."

"Okay, awesome. Thank you."

"Okay James, we are waiting for the Pre-Anesthesia team to be ready for you. Then, we will move you over to that room. I want to wish you luck this morning!"

"Thank you."

HOPE WITHIN ME

A man walked into the room, not long after the nurse explained everything to me, and wheeled my bed over to Pre-Anesthesia. Once I was there, my bed was pushed into a bed spot. There were multiple beds and people in the room. Multiple nurses came in and gave me intravenous lines, took my blood pressure, and checked my oxygen level. I waited in the room for an hour. There had been a clock in front of my bed, so I stared at it for what seemed like forever. It was seven o'clock by the time part of my anesthesia team came in to talk to me.

"Good morning James." A young man said.

"Good morning."

" I will be your lead anesthesiologist today. Right here beside me will be my trusty second-hand anesthesiologist." Another young woman stood next to him. Both of them no older than thirty years old.

"Hello James." She smiled and waved. "There will also be a few others in your anesthesiology room as well, learning and watching."

"Okay." I nodded.

"The two of us will be back in a bit to take you over. But, first, did the nurses apply the sticky buttocks pads?" The young man asked.

"Yes, they did."

"Awesome. The neurosurgeon should be coming in before we take you, so hold on tight. See you in a bit James." He said. They both waved and left.

After both of the anesthesiologists had left, a nurse walked over to me. She wanted to know if I needed to use the bathroom or anything else before it was time for surgery since I was going to be in the operation for approximately four hours. I told her I didn't. After she had asked me, she told me I was able to remove my face mask, since it had been a sterile, disposable one the hospital gave me. I was more than glad to.

At seven twenty-five o 'clock, I saw a familiar face enter the Pre-Anesthesia room. It was Doctor Boden.

"Good morning James. How are you feeling this morning?"

"I'm doing alright."

"Good. I just want to come over and check in on you. I also want to take a look at your head. I am going to mark where we are going to enter in at." With a marker, he drew an X over my right ear, which is where my right Temporal Lobe is located. "Alright James, everything looks good." He walked around my bed. "They have your intravenous lines ready, so I'll see you in the operation room." He walked out of the room.

The two anesthesiologists walked in again.

"Hi James, are you ready. We heard Doctor Boden just left and it looks like he marked your head already." The young man said.

"Yeah, he did."

"So, we are going to take you over to your anesthesia room now."

HOPE WITHIN ME

I was wheeled out to a private room where there was a metal table in the center. I was lifted up onto the metal table by the two anesthesiologists as well as the team that had been waited in the room. I was laid flat on my back on the cold metal. Again, there was a clock centered in front of the table. I started to get scared. My mind raced with thoughts and things that could possibly happen. The risks of the operation were slim, but I knew the chances as well.

I could die. I might never see my family again. Days before the operation, I had switched my beneficiaries over to my sisters. I wanted them to always be taken care of if something happened to me. *At least I know my sisters will be okay for a while if something happens.* I stared at the clock, *Seven forty-six o'clock.*

"Okay James." The young man put a mask on my face. "This is just oxygen right now. Just breath in and out like normal."

I was terrified. It was almost silent in the room other than the stream of oxygen that went through the tube. I wanted to cry, but I knew I wasn't able to. I felt so alone, so cold.

I want to go home. I don't know if I want to do this anymore. God please, I'm so scared right now. I feel so alone. Please protect me.

The young woman walked over to me, "Okay, start taking deep breaths in and out now."

I started to take deeper breathes. I looked at her to make sure I was doing okay.

"Good job. We are going to switch it over to the anesthesia now, but keep taking those nice, deep breathes." The man said.

JAMES VALENCIA

I stared at the clock that sat on the wall in front of me. While I took deeper breathes, I started to feel weird. The young man walked over to me.

"James, you're doing great. You see these lines right here?" He pointed to lines that dipped lower each time I took a breath. "that means the anesthesia is working."

I spent the rest of the time looking at the clock, *Seven fifty-three o'clock.*

God, I'm so scared right. I wish I were home and with my family. Whatever happens next, I trust and hope it's for the better. If I don't make it out of this operation and die, at least I'll finally be with You. Please God, I'm so scared. I really don't want to be here right now. Please.

A NEW DAY – WEDNESDAY JULY 15, 2020

I woke up in the *Intensive Care Unit* later that evening on Tuesday July 14, for what seemed like

only a few minutes before I fell asleep again. I was dazed and groggy from the anesthesia and the

surgery, so I didn't know what time it was. I stayed in the *Intensive Care Unit* for one night only.

Still groggy from the procedure, I was woken up the next day, Wednesday July 15, by nurses

who had shoved a board under me so they could transfer me from one bed to another. Once I was

transferred to the new bed, I was wheeled out of the *Intensive Care Unit* and taken down

multiple hallways to a different room. Once I was in the room, my bed was lowered, and my

intravenous lines were connected to everything. It was hard for me to wake up, but from what I

saw when I looked around, I recognized the room. It was the room I had done my Video EEG

monitoring in back in May. I knew I must have been on floor nine, Adult Neurology.

I slept most of the day, but by the time I was able to try and sit up, I looked around for my bag. I knew the nurse down in the Pre-Operation room had said it was going to follow me. A nurse had seen me sit up, so she came and assisted me.

"Do you need help with anything James?"

"I was wondering where my bag was, that's all."

"Hmm...that's a good question. Let me check with the nurse's station. Also, how is your pain level right now?"

"My head hurts a lot. It's also hard for me to talk and move my jaw."

"Yeah, it will be like that for a few days, but it will get better. I can go and get you some pain medication right now."

She left and brought back my bag and some extremely strong pain medication.

"Here is your bag, it was sitting at the nurse station, and some pain medication. Whenever your head starts to hurt, let me know and I'll try to give you some if I can." She handed me a cup of water and pills.

I checked my phone once she left the room. I had several messages from family, friends, and professors. I replied to every message, as I was touched that so many people had thought about me that morning and throughout the day of the operation. Not long after going through the messages, lunch arrived at my room. The nurse brought it into my room.

"Hi James, lunch is here. So, we have soft foods for you to eat. When you eat, try not to open your mouth and jaw too much. If you do it will start to hurt where they did the operation. Chew lightly and slowly, okay. Let me know if you need help"

"Okay, I will. Thank you." I started to eat once she left.

I tried not to open my jaw so much, but at times I did, and ended up hurting myself. I constantly reminded myself to chew slow and to be careful. The slightest movement of my head or body made my head hurt. Later that evening, I received a surprise visit from Doctor Boden.

"Hello James, how are you feeling?"

"I'm okay. I'm just in a lot of pain."

"Yeah, we prescribed you some strong medication to help with your pain when you go home. As well as some steroids for brain swelling, which happens anytime the brain is touched."

"Okay."

"You look good though. Your procedure went very well. It took a little over three and a half hours to complete. The tools and tactics we used were microdissection, so we could see clearly, stereotactic navigation, so we could be sure to get all of it out in a safe and effective way, and we used a normal blade we normally would use for this type of operation."

"That's good to hear."

"Also, we removed part of your skull, cleaned it, and after the procedure, sutured it back in place. So, it is still your original bone, no metal. You have nylon sutures though, not dissolvable ones. So those will need to be removed in a couple of weeks."

"Okay, so I will make any appointment for that?"

"Yes, in about two weeks. I will get you a referral for that."

"Okay."

"The exciting part of the operation was that we removed all of the encephalocele, all **3mm** of it. I will leave you to rest now and I will get those referrals ready. Your operation was remarkably successful James. You should be happy."

"Thank you Doctor Boden."

Doctor Boden and the team that was with him, which I only guessed was in the operating room at the time, left my room. The nurse walked back into the room.

"Hi James, are you all done with your lunch?"

"Yes I am."

"How are you feeling now? Any pain?"

"I feel better. It still hurts and it's hard to move, but not as much pain."

"Well, you did just have brain surgery, so it will take some getting used to."

"Yeah, I guess you're right."

"Not everyone can say they've had it, or else everyone would be having it. You're strong for going through it James. Think about it, now you can officially say you have had brain surgery." She tried to cheer me up.

She grabbed my tray. "Also, Doctor Boden says if you're doing well enough, and we can get you walking soon, you might be able to go home by Thursday or Friday."

"Okay."

"How are you feeling? Do you think you can walk? If not, no worries."

"Can I try to walk today?"

"Sure. Let me go set this tray down and get another nurse to help."

She went to grab another nurse and came back to unhook me from the machines in the room. I put on the hospital socks for grip, and I slowly put my legs to one side of the bed. Each of the nurses held my arms as I tried to lift myself up and out of the bed. As I rose from the bed, my head started to hurt.

"Alright James, how is your head feeling?"

"It hurts a little now, but I think it's because I was laying down for so long."

"Yeah, it's because you have liquid in your brain right now. As you walk, move, and urinate, the drainage from the swelling in your brain will go away."

"Okay."

"For now, let's walk to the nurse's station." We walked. "How are you feeling? You think you can go farther, or back to the room?"

"I think I can do more walking."

"Alright, let's go!" We walked around the nurse's station and through the *Epilepsy Monitoring Unit* before we headed back to the room. All of the staff waved and smiled to me.

"Very good job today James. You did excellent walking today. Let me check for outward drainage really quick." She checked my incision for any leaks. "Good, nothing. Keep drinking water, juice, and any liquid so that the swelling goes down. I think you're ready to go home and heal there tomorrow."

I was happier than ever to hear that I was able to go home so soon. I wanted to see my family and be in my own bedroom. I knew what I had experienced opened my eyes to a new way of life. I knew I needed to begin healing, emotionally and physically.

. . . . .

Thursday July 16, the nurse came into my room.

"Good morning James. I have your AEDs, as well as pain medication." She handed me a cup filled with colorful pills.

"When will I be able to go home?"

"We are getting your discharge papers ready right now. Before you go, do you think you can walk around one more time?"

"Yes."

She helped me get out of the bed and stand up again. We walked the same route we had the day before. We walked the *Epilepsy Monitoring Unit* before I was back in the bed.

"Okay James, great job. Once your discharge papers are ready, you are all set. Do you have a ride? We will be taking you down in a wheelchair"

"Yes. I will text them right now. Before you go, can I use the bathroom please?"

"Yes, since you are walking really good, you can use the regular bathroom and not the container." I was helped up again and I walked to the bathroom.

When I walked into the bathroom, I saw myself in the mirror for the first time. I walked closer to the mirror and turned my head. It was scabbed and bloody. I looked awful, ugly. I had a giant scar on the side of my head. It was the shape of a backwards question mark, about the size of the palm of my hand. I cried in the bathroom. I kept looking at the scar and remembered all of the torture it had brought me throughout half of my life. I cried at the shame I felt again. Then, I remembered, there was hope. That it had all happened for a reason, and that I had to wait for it to work and let the past be the past.

Once I was finished using the bathroom, I washed my hands and walked out to the bed. The nurse came in and went over the discharge papers and medications.

"Is your ride here yet James?"

I looked at my phone. "Yes, they are waiting in the parking lot."

"Okay, awesome. Are you ready to go home then and be comfortable?"

"Yeah."

A wheelchair was brought into the room, and I sat down in it. I was wheeled down to the lobby of the *Medical Center* before I was brought out front. My father waited in the car, and the nurse helped me stand up and into the car.

I was glad to be on my way home. Those had been three long days for me, and I was still depressed about how I looked with the giant scar. The scar reminded me of everything I had been through. But I knew I needed to keep my faith that the surgery had worked. That even if it didn't plan out the way I had hoped, it was all going to be okay. But for the time being, I had to keep believing.

When I arrived home, my mother couldn't have been happier to see me. We hugged each other and talked about the hospital stay. I explained to both of my parents how I needed to rest and heal. I also explained what Doctor Boden had told me in the room. My father went out later that evening to get soft foods for me to eat while I recovered. I was glad to be home that day.

V

. . . . .

Even the darkness is not dark to You, and the night is

as bright as the day. Darkness and light are alike to You.

PSALM 139:12

But those who hope in the Lord will renew their strength. They

will soar on wings like eagles; they will run and not grow

weary, they will walk and not be faint.

ISAIAH 40:31

V

HEALING BEGINS

I woke up on Friday July 17, and I was back at home in my bedroom in my own bed. It felt nice, it felt comfortable. I knew I needed to heal at that point. I had all of the discharge instructions and papers that described how to do so physically, however, the hardest part of all of it would be how to do so emotionally. I had to believe and continue to have the faith and hope I had prior to the surgery in order for my healing to work.

After so many days of eating soft foods, I had gotten used to it. Although it had started to get boring at times, I had sucked it up for a while longer until I was able to open my jaw wider without it hurting. I knew it was going to be like that for a while, so I had to make the best of it, which I did. About four days after discharge, I was able to start cleaning the incision, so my mother helped with that. It became a routine every night, where I was to go downstairs before bed and she would clean the incision very gently for me. We cleaned it with antibacterial soap and warm water with our fingers, so the scabs were not removed. Then, we applied ointment, that kept from infections from forming.

I had started to have hearing and vision problems a few days post-surgery, so I called neurosurgery and informed them. They told me it was normal and if it continued to call them in two weeks. They said it was the brain trying to adjust to everything as it had just undergone a major operation. I kept my hopes high, but it had gotten extremely hard.

NEW NORMAL

I had been having a difficult time adjusting to life. My thoughts and brain were everywhere at the time, and everything felt different. I had not forgotten anything, but the perspective in which I saw things had changed due to the operation and it felt strange to me. I knew I had to just let my brain do its own thing and adjust. Nothing felt right or normal, but I was soon to have a *New Normal*.

Before the operation, Doctor Boden, and Doctor Devrat had warned me that I needed to prepare myself emotionally for the change post-surgery. That everyone who had the operation experienced not just the physical aspect of losing a piece of their brain, but also the "normal life" that had been associated with it. The normal that had been a part of my life for so long, had started to fade, and a *New Normal* had started to take form. However, I didn't know how to cope with the reality of it. When Doctor Boden and Doctor Devrat had told me about the *New Normal* I would encounter, they had told me there was no way to describe it. It was something I needed to prepare myself for emotionally when the time came post-operation. The way my brain had started to adjust at that point scared me as it had started to adjust daily. I constantly tried to look forward to a new future ahead, but at the same time was constantly reminded of a traumatized past.

FRIENDS – JULY 25, 2020

I had still been trying to cope with adjusting to my *New Normal* when I received a phone call on

a Tuesday morning. I looked at my phone, and it was a number and name that had made me

happy to see, it was my friend from college, Ted. I answered my phone.

"Hello?"

"Hey, Jimmy!"

"Hey Tedd." I laughed, hurting my jaw a bit. Something I hadn't done in a while though.

"What are you up to?"

"Nothing, I'm just at home watching television. What about you?"

"I'm doing the same thing. Darla is with me too." Darla was Ted's girlfriend who he had

met our junior year of college.

"Hey Jimmy!" Darla yelled in the background.

"Hi Darla."

"Darla and I just wanted to know if you wanted to hangout for a little. We wanted to visit you since you just had surgery and buy you dinner."

"Sure. Uh, what time? You live like forty minutes away."

"We don't mind the drive; we just want to see how you are doing. We can be there by three o' clock?"

"Yeah, that works. You still have my address?"

"Yeah, I sure do man."

"Cool, I'll see you in a bit then. Bye Ted."

"Bye Jimmy."

"Bye Darla!" I yelled so she was able to hear me.

It had been nice that my friends wanted to see me. I needed a "pick-me-up" since I was an emotional wreck at the time. I was excited to see them though, *I just hope they don't mind my scar*, that's all I had thought to myself.

Later that day, I received a text message from Tedd. They were passing the Liberal Arts College, where all three of us had gone to school. The college was only four miles away from where I lived, so I needed to get ready. I quickly went up to my bedroom, changed my shirt and went back downstairs and waited. Again, had received another phone call, however that time it came from Darla.

"Hey Darla."

"Jimmy! We are here."

I went to the front door and they stood right there. We greeted each other with giant hugs before we all walked into the house. We sat down in the living room and talked for a while before we went outside and sat down.

"So, Jimmy, how have you been?" Ted asked.

"I've been good. Just trying to adjust to everything."

"Has it been hard? Does it feel different?" Darla asked next.

"It does feel different, but I remember everything. It's just been a new way of living basically which is weird to me. But it's hopefully for the better, you know?"

"Yeah, definitely. You were having so many seizures." Ted said.

"We are so happy for you though. We hope this all works!" Darla said with a smile.

"Me too. I think it will, it will just take some time. How have you two been though?

"Good. Just stuck at home with this virus and this global pandemic." Ted and Darla looked at each other and shook their heads. "We've been bored."

"Yeah, I think everyone has, honestly."

After we had talked, we decided to go to a little Mexican food place to get food. I ordered a bean burrito, as I needed something soft I was able to eat, and Ted and Darla ordered tacos. We

JAMES VALENCIA

had ordered the food to go and brought it back to where I lived. We spent an hour that day

reminiscing about college, and our trips when we studied abroad, Ted and I in Salzburg, Darla in

London. We talked about the fraternity and how we used to hang out with friends and drink, or

how we were late to class and how we liked or didn't like certain professors. So many good

memories from the past, it had felt like so long ago in that moment.

It had started to get dark soon after we finished dinner, and Ted and Darla didn't want to

drive back home in the dark, as their drive was forty minutes. So, I said my good-byes to them.

"Bye Jimmy." Ted hugged me. "We will hopefully see you soon again."

"Yes, hopefully we will see each other soon. Bye Ted. Be safe driving."

"Bye Jimmy." Darla hugged me as well.

"Bye Darla."

The two of them walked out of the house and drove away. We waved to each other until

they were gone. It had felt nice that the two of them had come to visit. It made me feel normal

again. It made that day special, made me happy again. An emotion I hadn't felt in a long time.

. . . . .

July 26, I had decided to contact my friend Jeff who I had gone to college with. We

talked over video chat on our laptops. He lived in Arizona, so his version of the pandemic was

276

different than California's as regulations in our country varied somewhat. After we talked for about an hour about life, and how I had been doing, and what he had been up to we ended the call.

However, not long after the call had ended that day, I felt the feeling. It was back. I felt the feeling I usually felt before I had a seizure. It was a small rising sensation, but not the full thing. It stopped before it had actually begun. And there had been no seizure. There was no actual aura either. It had been the weirdest thing. I had started to get scared. I was confused as to what it *actually* was. At that point, I had really been worried whether or not the surgery had worked. Whether all of the pain and emotional damage had been worth it. I needed to wait and find out.

NO MORE SUTURES - THURSDAY JULY 30, 2020

It was a Thursday and I had felt defeated at that point. Four days prior, I had felt the same feeling

I had used to feel before surgery. My emotions were all over the place, but, on that day I was

happy. I had gotten ready to go to a neurosurgery follow-up appointment to get the sutures they

had used to stitch up my head removed. I went to the same building where I had the original

appointment with Doctor Boden and went through the same routine I went through multiple

times throughout the five months before. I was stopped at the door, my temperature was checked,

received a clearance to enter, given a sterile face mask, checked in, and sat down in the waiting

area. Though that time when I had gone to the appointment, it had felt different. It may have

been from the surgery and my adjusting to the *New Normal*, or that I was nervous to get the

sutures removed that day. Either way, I waited alone in the waiting area until I was called to go to a back room. The follow up had been with one of Doctor Boden's assistant's, not actually him.

"Hello James, how are you doing today?" The assistant asked.

"I'm doing good. How are you?

"I'm well. I just want to go over some questions with you about your head."

"Okay."

"Have you been getting any headaches, nausea, lightheadedness, etc.?"

"No."

"Good. How about vision or hearing problems?"

"Well, actually yeah. I called about a week and a half ago about that."

The assistant checked my eyes, then looked in my ears for signs of any problems.

"It looks like you have a small ear infection."

"What does that mean for me? Is that bad for my brain?"

"No, not at all. I will prescribe you some medication and it should go away in about three to four weeks. That should also help the vision."

"Okay." Part of me was relieved. He continued to ask me another question.

"Do you have any drainage problems with your incision from your brain?"

"No, I haven't had anything like that."

"Great. Alright James, let's remove those sutures then." He took a pair of what looked like metal looking plyers and one by one plucked each individual suture out of my head. My skull was numb, so I didn't feel a thing except for a little pressure and pulling when he took the sutures out. It had been the weirdest thing to me.

"Okay James, you are all done. Now, I am going to give you a referral to make an appointment in October for your three-month follow-up MRI as well your follow-up with Doctor Boden."

"Okay."

"Make sure you give Doctor Boden at least one week to go over your MRI before your appointment with him. So, schedule the MRI first, a week in advance, and then schedule your appointment with Doctor Boden. You're all set."

"Okay, I will." I went to the front desk on my way out of the office and made the appointments for October.

By the end of that appointment, I was ready to leave and on my way home. It felt weird to not have the sutures in my head. It had even looked different. It was no longer puffy and looked somewhat normal. But I knew the scar was still there, which had bothered me. It was a transition I needed to adjust to over time.

FEELINGS

AUGUST had arrived and I still tried to adjust to my *New Normal* that I knew I needed to embrace. I had still been eating soft foods at that point but had slowly been progressing into harder foods which made me a somewhat happier person. But, in the back of my mind sat the thought of whether the operation had actually accomplished anything which still bothered me to my core.

· · · · ·

On August 3, I sat downstairs with my parents as we watched "trash" television one evening, as we always did. I had just finished dinner when I felt the feeling. Again, it wasn't the

283

full thing though. It was the feeling in my stomach before my aura, then it stopped within seconds. There had been no actual seizure from what I could tell. I was scared though. I looked over at my parents, then back at the television. I didn't know what to do, as I didn't want to tell them. I was afraid to tell them. Afraid that after all I had put them through, with the surgery, and waiting to see whether it was going to work out, they would be disappointed in the results. So, I kept it to myself. I went to bed that night and prayed it was nothing.

. . . . .

Four days after I had felt the feeling with my parents downstairs, I felt another one on August 7. I felt it in the afternoon, as I watched television in my bedroom. I ignored it at first, so I continued to watch whatever I had been watching.

Later that evening, I went downstairs and watched television with my parents like I usually did and felt another weird sensation. There was no aura or seizure from what I felt. My hope had dwindled, and I had become hopeless in the battle I thought I had overcome. Without a word spoken, I went up to my bedroom, and laid on my bed. I wondered whether life would get easier or if I was destined to live a life trapped in whatever I had been experiencing.

. . . . .

HOPE WITHIN ME

On August 12, I decided to get up early to make breakfast. My parents had both gone to work, and everyone in the house was still asleep. As I got dressed for the day, there it was again. The feeling. When would it end. My hope and faith that had grown so strong up until that point barely hung by a thread. I was tired and exhausted of the journey. I had been through so much pain and disappointment through the years, I didn't think I could have borne anymore.

. . . . .

It was August 21, a Friday morning, when my father and I decided to go visit my uncle and aunt for breakfast. I was excited, as I had not seen anyone in my family since before the operation, and with all of the feelings I had been experiencing at the time, it was nice to see people. We met my uncle at a small Mexican takeout place and ordered food to go, as there were no sit-down places due to the global pandemic. We took it back to their house, where we met up with my aunt, who worked from home, again due to the virus that ravaged our world at the time. Afterwards, we talked and laughed.

"Hey mijo, how does it feel to have that scar on your head? Does it feel different?" My uncle asked.

"A little. I'm still getting used to it."

"Do you remember things? Do you remember me, and this house?" My uncle joked.

"Yeah, I do." I laughed.

My aunt came downstairs to eat, as she was on her break from work.

"Hey Jimmy." She gave me a hug. "Wow, your head looks great. Once your hair grows back you won't even be able to tell there's a scar there." When she said that, it made me happy. I had been self-conscious every time I left the house or had gone anywhere in public.

"That's what I'm hoping."

My aunt and uncle gave my dad and I a tour of their house. They had just remodeled most of it at the time. They had repainted, recarpeted, new backsplash in their kitchen, new countertops, new doors, new lights, everything. It was beautiful.

Soon, my aunt went back upstairs to her office to work, and my uncle, dad, and I sat on the couches in their living room. We talked for a while, but halfway through the talking I felt the feeling. That feeling I felt was a different feeling then the rest. It was an awful feeling, as it felt like the auras I used to have when I had seizures. My dad and uncle continued to talk, and I sat on the couch, as I embraced it with my two hands in case I did have a seizure. I waited. I felt the rising sensation start in my stomach and make its way up through my upper body and through my chest. I was terrified, I didn't know what to do. I thought for sure I was going to have a seizure, but by the time it made it to my chest the sensation stopped. I had been a little shaky afterwards, but there was no seizure, only the aura-like feeling. I knew I needed to call the neurology or neurosurgery office as soon as possible when I arrived home that day.

HOPE WITHIN ME

When my father and I arrived home that day, I called neurology. No one answered. I left a message and described what had occurred. I was scared that day but told no one. The only one who knew was me and God. I prayed it wouldn't happen again.

. . . . .

On Saturday August 22, the day after my father and I visited with my uncle and aunt, we were headed to the grocery store. My father had forgotten something in the house and asked me to go get it. So, I had willingly gone to get it. On my way out, as he waited in the car and I closed the door to the house, I froze. I felt the feeling again. The feeling I had felt the day prior. I felt the rising sensation go through my upper body. I grabbed onto something in case I fell. But, again, it stopped. No seizure, only what had felt like an aura. I couldn't tell if it had actually been an aura or not though. I continued out to the car and my father and I went to the store. I was confused.

. . . . .

I sat downstairs with my mother on August 24 and watched television. I started to get a heavy feeling in my body though, which was a feeling I had never felt before. With my phone in

287

hand, which weighed maybe half a pound, it started to get heavy. It started to feel like five pounds, then ten. I looked around the room at my mother, as my father had gone to bed already. The room started to close in and get heavy. Pressure came down on me. I didn't know how to react or feel. So, I stood up and walked to the kitchen and pretended to do things. I wanted to shake the feeling. The feeling soon ended, and I was confused. I said good night to my mother and went to my bedroom and tried to watch television there instead.

That evening as I watched television in my bedroom, I was on my laptop shopping online. Again, the same feeling returned. The room came down on me. The pressure was heavy, the laptop became heavy too. I lifted my hand that time and it was hard to lift as it felt like it was fifty pounds. I was scared. I stood up again and tried to shake the feeling. I waited for it to end. As it ended, I changed into my pajamas, and tried to sleep it off by watching television. I eventually turned the television off and just stared at my ceiling. I thought of all the hope and faith I had throughout the year. I still had it, but it was hard for me to believe. I didn't know what was happening to me at the time. *Was this my New Normal?* I was confused. I wanted answers.

God, I can't go through this anymore. I've gone through over ten years of this struggling. Half of my life has been taken from me. How much longer must I suffer and go through this pain and torture? Make it end, please. I'm tired and exhausted. I need you to help me. This burden is too much for me to bear anymore. Please. Show yourself to me in ways I never imagined.

EMERGENCY APPOINTMENT – TUESDAY AUGUST 25, 2020

The first thing I did the following morning, as everyone had gone to work or left for the day, was called the neurology office. I was desperate for answers. Was I in fact having auras or seizures unknowingly, or was this my *New Normal* I needed to adjust to? When I called the neurology office at the *Medical Center*, Doctor Devrat's nurse answered the phone.

"Hi James, how are you doing this morning?" She asked me right away.

"I'm not sure, I have a few issues."

"Okay, what's going on?"

"Ever since I had my craniotomy, I've been having really weird feelings."

"Can you describe them to me so I can take note of them?"

"Yeah. They feel almost like the beginning of the auras I used to have before my seizures but not quite like them either."

"When did they start, how many do you think you've had, and how often are they occurring?"

"The first one was on July 26, then I've had six more after that. All within three to five days a part. It's really worrying me now."

"Okay, that's a total of seven in a month since your surgery. So, what I'm going to do is schedule you an appointment to see Doctor Devrat today if I can. Let me look at his schedule right now."

"Okay, thank you."

She looked through his schedule, and I prayed there was an opening available.

"Okay sweetheart, he has an opening at two o 'clock this afternoon. Does that work for you?"

"Yes, that would be perfect!"

"Alright, he will see you online at two then. Bye James."

"Bye." I hung up the phone.

I hoped that appointment was going to give me some sort of answer or reassurance to what was happening to me and my brain. That whatever laid ahead for me, was a good thing.

It had been exactly six weeks since the operation on my brain by that point, so after I had talked on the phone I decided I was going to go on my very first "exercise walk" outside. The instructions for healing I had been given stated that I was not allowed to exercise for a minimum

of four to six weeks. So, to be safe, I waited the full six weeks. I had been used to exercising

almost every day prior to the craniotomy, so just sitting at home had made me feel awful.

I put on my walking shoes and stepped onto the front porch. It was a cool morning, and I

was nervous and anxious to get out there. I knew I had to go slow though. The *Medical Center*

had instructed me to walk slow and take breaks if my head started to hurt, which were signs I had

over exhausted my body and brain. I went really slow that morning, which I hadn't been used to.

But there was a smile on my face the entire time I walked. I took multiple breaks, not because

my head had hurt, but to be safe for myself and brain. By the time I had returned home, I was the

happiest I had been in a long time. I had tracked my distance and time. It came out to one third of

a mile and twenty-five minutes. It had been the slowest I had ever gone, but I knew it was going

to take time to build back up to where I used to be.

After the walk that day, I waited for the neurology appointment. I was happy I had

scheduled one. I hoped and had faith there was an answer to my problems I had been having.

By the time two o'clock came around that day it was time to call the neurology office on

my laptop.

"Good morning James, how are you doing today?" Doctor Devrat asked.

"I'm doing alright."

"I hear you are having problems. Can you describe them to me?"

"So, I've been having the same feelings I had during my auras when I had a seizure. But they aren't quite like the full aura. I don't know if that makes any sense."

"Describe the feelings to me. Any smells, tingling, vision loss, etc.?"

"The first one, on July 26, was the feeling in my stomach like my old aura but it stopped after maybe a second or two. The second one, on August 3 felt the exact same way. It started in my stomach but stopped. However, on August 7, I had two weird feelings."

"Describe August 7 to me. What did those feel like? And what were you doing?" Doctor Devrat took notes as I talked and described my feelings.

"On August 7, the first feeling I felt I was watching television in my bedroom. Again, the same feeling as the first few. The second feeling that day I was downstairs with my family watching television in the evening."

"Okay James, and the nurse said you had few more feelings than just these?"

"Yes, I also had a feeling in the morning on August 12 as I got dressed for the day. Also, I had a few scarier ones."

"Tell me about the scarier ones James."

"On August 21, I was at my uncle and aunt's house when I felt what I thought was a full aura. Like, the full rising sensation from my stomach through my upper body. I was sitting on their couch, so I clutched onto it and braced for what I thought was going to be a seizure. But then it stopped. It really scared me. That exact feeling happened again the following day on

August 22 when I was walking out of the front door of my house. The same rising sensation. I thought for sure I was going to have a seizure. And on August 24, I sat with my mother downstairs and watched television when I got a heavy feeling in my body."

"Describe August 24 to me."

"I was sitting on the couch holding my phone, and it started to get heavy. It felt like it weighed five or maybe ten pounds. It was very strange to me."

"Did it feel like the room was closing in on you?"

"Yeah, that's a good way of describing it. Everything just felt heavy. The air, the room, my whole body. I eventually got up to walk around and it went away. I then went up to my bedroom to watch television and go shopping online on my laptop. And the same thing happened. I don't know what that feeling was, I had never felt it before."

"Okay James, interesting feelings. So, the good news is, you were able to describe every detail incredibly clear to me. Something you weren't able to do before."

"What does that mean?" I was confused. I had just wanted to know if I had a seizure or not.

"It means, you are no longer having Focal Onset Impaired Awareness Seizures. As in, your awareness is no longer impaired. That's an extremely good thing for you and tells us the surgery has done its' job up to this point."

"Okay. What about the feelings though?"

"The feelings could be anything. It could be possible that your brain is still adjusting to things as it has only been..." He counted aloud, "a month, not even two yet. Your brain needs time to adjust. Or, it could mean you are having Focal Onset Aware Seizures."

"Focal Onset Aware Seizures? What does that mean?" The thought of another type of seizure stressed me out.

"Focal Onset Aware Seizures mean that you are fully conscious and able to do things during the seizure. It doesn't inhibit your motor abilities or consciousness like when you would have your Impaired Awareness Seizures. If that's the case, that is still progress James. You should be happy, as you described a lot of information to me today that you never would have been able to before surgery."

"So, what do we do from here then? Will they go away if they are Focal Onset Aware Seizures?"

"Try not to stress about it because your brain is still healing. It's only been a month out since the operation. The operation doesn't guarantee one-hundred percent seizure free. But we are confident your brain will adjust with time. Give it time James. How is your environment and stress level?"

"I've actually been really stressed lately. Most of it coming from whether or not the surgery worked. I noticed I've been shaky too. I'll hold my hand out in front of me, and it shakes. I think I have a lot of anxiety about this."

HOPE WITHIN ME

"Yeah, we need to do something to control the electrical current in your brain. I'm going to prescribe you an anti-anxiety medication called *Clonazepam*. It will make you sleepy, so I want you to take it at bedtime. They will be 0.5mg tablets, just take one every night. This should help reduce your anxiety and stress. But really, try to monitor your stress, and try not to worry about the surgery. It's doing great so far. The surgery went extremely well, and the results are showing even a month out."

"Okay. I'll try not to worry so much and stress about it."

"If you do have any more feelings, keep track of them. I will send you a referral so I can see you again in a couple of months."

"Okay. Thank you Doctor Devrat."

"Alright James. You're doing great. Bye now."

We hung up our calls that afternoon . I was still worried, but knew I needed to lower my stress level. I was happy I had received the anti-anxiety medication though. I knew it was going to help me. But I also knew I needed to put in some work as well. I knew going on walks, listening to relaxing music, and meditating were ways to help as well. I needed to turn my worries into something positive for my own sake if I wanted it all to work.

295

SELF-CARE – FALL 2020

As fall arrived that year, my stress level started to decrease slowly, partially due to the new anti-anxiety medication. I had also started to meditate and read books before bed instead of watching television. I started to listen to more soothing classical music in my spare time, as well as exercise on a regular basis again which had made me feel confident. I was determined, but not stressed, to find new ways to live out a lifestyle that would be more beneficial to my overall mental and emotional health.

With that, came the daunting realization of depression. One I never thought I had been in until that fall. By the time I realized I was depressed, it was August 27. The more I thought about it, I knew it had come from the surgery, having lived with Epilepsy for over ten years and struggling with a battle I never thought I would win. I still had the constant fear of everything falling apart, but as Doctor Devrat had said two days earlier at the august 25 appointment, I needed to be confident in myself.

On that day, I made a choice I never regretted. I went to a supply store, bought a plastic box, a photo album, a journal, and folders. I put all of my Epilepsy information inside of that box. Inside the photo album I started to place pictures of my scar from the craniotomy. I took a picture every week, put the picture with a label in the photo album, and would continue until the one-year anniversary of the operation to see the progress as a memory of how I had overcome one of the greatest battles of my life. The journal, I had started to journal every week, just once, to write down feelings. Whether good or bad, just so they didn't bottle up. In the folders, I placed every single document, referral, and test result ever given to me, pre-surgery/appointment and post-surgery/appointment dated back to 2019. I labeled the box *My Epilepsy Story: My Right Temporal Lobe Craniotomy w/ Epileptogenic Focus*. I placed the box on my bookshelf where I only pull it out to put pictures, documents, and journal once a week.

After I created the Epilepsy Box for myself, I also decided I wanted to rent a baby grand piano. I don't know what made me want to rent a piano, but something, maybe it was how I missed music, as it had always been a part of me, but I rented a beautiful mahogany baby grand piano. It was delivered on August 30 to my home. I played on the piano every day when I was able to that fall. My depression started to fade away, and once again, I saw hope in my future.

EPILEPSY ADVOCATE

As I started to become a happier person, I had found ways to do so. And in September, I was interested in how to participate with the *Epilepsy Foundation of America* and other Epilepsy organization events. One way in which I found out in doing so was to be a part of the *Epilepsy Foundation of America's, Walk to End Epilepsy*. Due to the virus pandemic, it was a virtual walk that fall. So, I joined the Southern California and Northern California walks. I also joined another Epilepsy organization's walk they presented. I signed up for all three virtual walks on September 1. I was excited, as I had never advocated before. As someone who had lived with the chronic illness for over ten years, I wanted to support and give a hope to people.

· · · · ·

On September 19, I had the first virtual walk. It was with the small Epilepsy organization from Northern California. Luckily, everything was virtual, so I walked early in the morning that day. After I had walked, I came back home where I logged onto my laptop and onto a video chat with everyone. We had all been given a link to login. We talked for an hour about our walks, how far we walked, why we walked, who we walked for, and where we were from. It was an incredible experience that day. I realized I was meant to advocate for people like myself and those who still battled Epilepsy. A few days after the walk, I received a t-shirt in the mail that read *Epilepsy Warrior*.

. . . . .

As the next couple of advocacy walks approached, I received an email, that was probably sent to everyone who had signed up for the walks, that asked a question. The question struck a personal part of my core. I stared at the question as I teared up and just thought about the answer I would give for it. The question had been: *What Would You Tell Your Younger Self? Looking back on when you or your loved one was diagnosed with Epilepsy...what words of encouragement and advice would you give yourself?* I stared for a while before I went to my Epilepsy Box, pulled out my journal, and wrote the question. After I reflected for as long as I could, I gave an answer. I cried the entire time as I wrote, before I set my pen down:

HOPE WITHIN ME

What Would You Tell Your Younger Self? Looking back on when you or your loved one was diagnosed with Epilepsy...what words of encouragement and advice would you give yourself?

Looking back to when I was first diagnosed with Epilepsy, I did not quite know what Epilepsy was or even a seizure was. I also thought the doctors knew everything about my condition and could fix it with medication. I soon found out that was not the case. I was even told soon after, that they had even heard of some children and teenagers "growing out of it" by their 20's. My family and myself thought for years that is what would happen. I almost feel like I was trying to convince myself I would "grow out of them". But soon, I was going through many medications, 6 by the end to be exact. Once college came around, I figured I would just need to find the right medication I could take for the rest of my life and I would be set. That was not the case for my type of Epilepsy I had. In 2019, 9 years after my diagnosis, my Epilepsy diagnosis was changed and diagnosed as Intractable Epilepsy.

I was asked if there was any advice I would give you, Jimmy, before or after I received the diagnosis in July of 2010. Some advice I would my 14-year-old self, would be to know that the doctors/specialists know what they are doing, but they are also learning as well about my specific type of Epilepsy/seizures, as seizures constantly change. Some Epilepsy/seizures become drug resistant where medication do not work, some people need devices implanted on their

301

brain, some people just need medication, and others need brain surgery. It just depends on their condition. Little did I know the journey I would go on would leave such a lasting mark on my life. So, 14-year-old self, be strong and resilient because you are strong. For what you will face will inspire many.

14-year-old self, if I give you a glimpse into what was to come, the same month you are diagnosed with Epilepsy (July 2010), exactly 10 years later (July 2020) you will be having a lobectomy for the removal of a 3mm piece of your right Temporal Lobe where the seizure focus is located. They found the focus of where all the seizure activity was coming from; however, it was still unknown what caused your Epilepsy.

Know that you are strong for what you are about to go through in the next 10 years. It will not be an easy road. There will be days throughout high school and college where you will cry out asking "Why?" or just sit somewhere to be alone. But know you make and meet so many friends and professors in college who love you until this very day and who are still with you and support you in all your endeavors. And know that God will be there every step of the way, even when it does not seem like it because there will be times it does, but He is there, I promise. On that surgery table, you will feel His presence the way I did.

I want you to know that you will become an inspiration to many of your friends and colleagues for your journey and all you will go through. They will rejoice with you, think of you, and send so much love to you. Also, one more thing, you will have a giant scar on the right side

HOPE WITHIN ME

of your head, and it will look like a giant question mark. It will be a reminder of all you have been through, your scars, your crying out for help and hope, your prayers, and your friends and family being there for you. But, most importantly of God's abundant love for you and how He has never left you during your journey with Epilepsy.

You are strong, brave, and have more courage than you will feel you have at the time of your diagnosis and in the journey, I promise you Jimmy.

As I finished writing my answer to that question, I closed the journal and sat in the quietness. I reflected on everything I had been through, I put the journal back into the Epilepsy Box and placed the box back on my bookshelf. At the same time, as I had put the answer into words and onto the pages, the burden and darkness that once filled my life for so long had been lifted off of my shoulders and washed out of me. I felt free. *If only I had been given those words when I was younger*, I thought, *maybe I wouldn't have been an angry person, hiding in the darkness only waiting for a glimpse of light.* I continued with that day, happier, more satisfied than ever. I played the piano, read books, and watched television. I was a new person.

And surely I am with you always,

to the very end of the age.

MATTHEW 28:20

303

POST – OPERATION

MAGNETIC RESONANCE IMAGING

On Saturday October 10, 2020, I had scheduled an appointment for a post-operation MRI.
Doctor Boden wanted to see how my brain had adjusted since the surgery. So, that Saturday
evening I went into the radiology clinic to have one done. I was nervous that day, as the area of
my skull that the operation had been done in was still numb and fragile, so I didn't know how it
would work with the cage around my head.

I walked into the radiology office around four o' clock in the afternoon, where I checked
in, received a sterile mask, and waited. Since the pandemic around the world started, it had
gotten worse, so as I waited, I noticed there were more seats blocked off and distanced so no one
could sit close to each other. I waited in the lobby of the clinic for over forty-five minutes, which
irritated me, but I tried to make the best of it. As I sat there, I had been texting my good friend

Mayra. She had gone to the Liberal Arts College with me and was one of my closest friends. We considered each other best friends. She had also been one of the first friends that texted me the morning of the operation. She reassured me that the MRI would be fine. Finally, I was called back for the MRI.

"James, follow me."

I stood up and followed a young lady.

"Here is a locker if you need to place anything inside. Just take out the key when you are done."

I placed everything in my pockets inside the locker. Then, I took off my belt and placed that inside as well, since that had metal on it. "Okay, I'm ready."

"Okay, I'll lead us to the MRI room then. Follow me." She said with a smile. We walked into a giant room with the MRI machine that sat inside. The bed had been pulled out already. "I will take the key you have and place it here on the ledge. Also, if you can remove your face mask since there is metal in it. No metal can go inside of the machine, it will pull it off your face."

"Okay." I handed her the face mask. I wasn't nervous since she had hers on still.

"Follow me, and we will place you on the machine bed James."

"Okay." We both walked over to the bed.

"Have you ever had an MRI before?"

I laughed a little at the question, "Yes, quite a few."

"Okay, that's good to know. Can I have you lay on the bed."

I laid down on the bed. As I did, I was careful with the right part of my head. "Oh, I had surgery a few months ago on my brain, so when you put the cage on my head could you be incredibly careful please? It's still very fragile."

"Oh wow. Yes, of course James."

"Thank you so much."

As she fitted the cage over my head, she put it on slow. "How is that? That doesn't hurt does it?"

"No, that's fine. Thank you." I smiled.

"Alright James, if you need anything push the button I am going to give you." She handed me the button. Then, she slid the bed into the MRI machine.

I laid there, with the cage fitted over my head. I stared at the blank whiteness of the tube. I tried to think of classical music and good memories. Then, suddenly I heard the sound. I felt the vibration the machine. The oh so familiar, loud, rhythmic sound of the MRI machine running its course as it captured images of my brain for the radiology technicians and Doctor Boden to review when it was finished.

After almost forty-five minutes of laying in the sound and vibration of the machine, it had stopped. My eyes had been closed, so I opened them not to know if it was finished or more pictures were to be taken. I finally heard footsteps in the room.

"Okay James, you are all done."

The bed started to move, and light appeared again. The lady smiled at me before she removed the cage from around my head.

"Good job today. And congratulations on a major surgery that you overcame."

"Oh, thank you." I smiled.

"So, we will review the images that we took today, and then send them to your doctor when we are finished. So give us and your doctor about four or five days to review everything."

"Okay. Thank you.

"Do you know how to exit the clinic from here? I know it's kind of large."

"Yes I do."

"Perfect. Just go back to the locker, grab your belongings, and leave the key. Then you are free to go. Bye James, have a great day."

"Bye." I grabbed my face mask before I walked out of the MRI room and to the locker where I had set down my belongings. I grabbed everything, and shoved them into my pockets, put my belt back on, and left the key in the locker again.

I left that appointment happy, as it had gone well. I only had to wait for the results and what Doctor Boden was going to find and say.

3 MONTH POST – OPERATION

NEUROSURGERY APPOINTMENT

Thursday October 22, 2020 I scheduled an appointment with Doctor Boden. I wanted to give him enough time to review the post-operation MRI Scan I had done the week prior. It had been a little over three months since the operation, so I was anxious to see him. When I arrived at the neurosurgery clinic that day, I waited to be called back. My hopes were somewhere in the middle, as I had been in the process of learning to trust it would all work out. As I waited for the nurse to call me back, I wondered what the conversation would look like that day. I had questions and things I wanted to tell Doctor Boden. So, I waited patiently that morning, as I knew there had been no appointment in front of mine, as I had booked the earliest appointment there was available that day with him. Finally, I was called back by one of Doctor Boden's nurses.

"James?"

"Hello." I smile at her and walked over to the door.

"Follow me sweetheart." She led me to a room. The same exact room where I had first met Doctor Boden back in June, and he told me I was a candidate for surgery. " Alright James, are all your medication on file correct?"

"Yes."

"Perfect. Doctor Boden will be with you shortly." She left the room.

I stared at the posters that hung on the wall. The same posters that I stared at almost four months earlier. My eyes were fixed on the one with the different lobes of the brain. *There it is. The right temporal lobe.* I thought to myself. I ran my fingers through my hair slowly and gently over my scar on the right side of my head. *Only, my temporal lobe is missing a 3mm piece now. Isn't that crazy?* I tried not to tear up as I felt my scar. I ran my index and middle finger along the entire length of the incision as I stared at the poster. I then heard a loud knock on the door of the room, and the door soon opened.

"Why hello James." A familiar face walked into the room, which broke my concentration on the poster.

"Hello." His presence made me happy.

"How are you feeling today?"

"I'm feeling good."

"Great." Doctor Boden logged into the computer in the room. "So, you did an MRI last week. Let's talk about that."

"Okay." I sat forward in the chair, nervous.

He showed me pictures of the MRI Scan on the computer screen. "Everything looks great. Your brain is adjusting normally and there seems to be no problems with symmetry. We can't find any abnormalities."

"That's good." I just stared at the screen.

"If you don't mind, James, can you turn your head so I can see your incision." He examined my incision and scar. "Your incision has healed very well for three months. Have you had any problems since the operation? Or do you have any questions?"

"Well, I was having quite a few Focal Onset Aware Seizures after the operation. I actually had a couple appointments with Doctor Devrat about it."

"With the Focal Seizures, what feelings did you feel?"

"It was a ton of déjà vu, lip tingling, even some feelings of my old auras. But I never had an actual old seizure that I used to have before surgery."

"Interesting. With the old feeling, what do you mean by that?"

"I had that feeling more after the operation. But it was the rising sensation from the mid body and up, but then it would stop. It never even felt like the full aura. It was weird."

"But did you ever lose consciousness like before?"

"No I never did."

"That's good."

"What about the Focal Onset Aware Seizures? Will those ever go away? I don't want to live with those."

"Sometimes we can't explain what these staring spells are. Sometimes they are something and sometimes they aren't. I think for you, you are progressing extremely well from the surgery and with time you will eventually be seizure free. You just need to not worry about it and let your brain adjust. Usually, when someone continues to have seizures after their surgery it is the exact same type of seizure they were having before the surgery. But for you that is not the case."

"Yeah, I think I was, and I am worrying too much. Doctor Devrat actually prescribed me an anti-anxiety medication because I had been shaky from stress from the surgery."

"I think it's time you relax, enjoy your life, and be confident in yourself. If you are confident that the surgery worked, your brain will adjust."

"Okay, I will be more confident in myself and the operation." I smiled.

"You look great James. Be confident in yourself." He walked me out to the lobby.

I left that appointment confident and happy. I knew deep inside of me and in my heart that I was going to be okay. I left with a giant smile.

The following was a review of Doctor Boden's Progress Notes from October 22, 2020:

HOPE WITHIN ME

SUBJECTIVE

James Valencia is a 24 y.o. male surgery patient for right temporal lobe Epilepsy 7/14/2020. After surgery he describes he has experienced spells of lip tingling and a recent episode he calls déjà vu consisting of a recollection of the prior epigastric auras he experienced prior to surgery. The tingling and déjà vu were not a part of his seizure pattern prior to surgery and he has had no loss of consciousness after surgery. Incision is well healed.

PAST SURGICAL HISTORY

PROCEDURE:	LATERALITY:	DATE:
Right temporal craniotomy for Epilepsy	Right	7/14/2020

2. Stereotactic Navigation 3. Microdissection

4. Resection of Epileptic Focus 5. Right

Corticoamygdalectomy 6. Cranioplasty

Performed by Doctor Boden, M.D. at Medical Center MAIN O.R.

ASSESSMENT:

Focal Onset Impaired Awareness Seizures, under excellent control. I think he is doing quite well and is and will be seizure free. He is very anxious, and he had benefited from the anti-anxiety medication prescribed by Doctor Devrat.

NEUROLOGY APPOINTMENT – FRIDAY OCTOBER 23, 2020

The day after the appointment with Doctor Boden, I had another three-month follow up

appointment scheduled with Doctor Devrat. I didn't need to go into the clinic that day, so I only

logged into my laptop early that morning for the video call with him. I was excited and nervous

at the same time when I saw him on the video call that day. He greeted me as he always did.

"Good morning James. Nice to see you."

"Good morning Doctor Devrat."

"How are you doing?

"I'm well. How about you?"

"I'm not bad. So, tell me, how are your feelings going? Have you had any more of

them?"

"Not since the last time that we spoke. I have had a few déjà vu feelings. But no more of the aura and rising sensations."

"That is very good to hear. With the déjà vu feelings, how often do you think you get them?"

"I would say probably one or two times a week at most. Is that bad?"

"Déjà vu is sometimes related to temporal lobe epilepsy and seizures. However, that is not always the case. Especially since you have been doing so well."

"So will I stop having them so frequently then?"

"It will take some time. Again, your brain is still adjusting James. Your brain has been living a certain way for ten years, and now it has stopped and needs to find a new way to live. That's very traumatic for it."

"Okay. I know when I saw Doctor Boden yesterday he told me I needed to be more confident in myself so my brain could adjust better. He said it would help my healing."

"Yes, he is absolutely right. I received a phone call from him yesterday afternoon about you, and he told me you looked and were healing great. Again, be confident in yourself and the surgery."

"Okay, I will be more confident." We both smiled. "So about the feelings?" I asked.

"So, those will go away with time. From what you and myself recorded, you haven't had an episode since August. That's a month and a half ago. That's great! And you haven't had a

Focal Onset Impaired Awareness Seizure since before the operation, that's even better. That means the surgery is working. What has happened is, your brain has so much scar tissue left over from all of the seizure activity you've had over the past nine to ten years. We call this Epileptic scar tissue that just sits on the brain, but this scar tissue will eventually go away with time as you don't have seizures."

"Okay." I tried to soak in as much information as I could. "Is that why all the déjà vu I'm having are memories from somewhat in that timeframe?"

"Your brain is remembering the traumatic portions it has been put through. But again if you are confident in yourself, your brain will adjust, and you will heal. Doctor Boden and I both believe you will be seizure free from this operation. Be confident in yourself and in the surgery. It's time to put this behind you and start living a normal life. You have a bright future ahead."

I smiled as he said that.

"Also James, since you have gone almost two months without a seizure now, it is still too early to lower your AEDs. However I want to go over the action plan with you."

"Okay." I was excited to hear his plan.

"We will start by lowering the *Zonisamide* first, since that is one of the newest ones. Then we will lower the *Lacosamide* next. How long have you been on the *Oxcarbazepine*?"

"That's one of the first AEDs I was ever given. So I'd say close to nine years now."

"Okay, so we will slowly lower that third since it has the highest dosage. So the goal is to have the *Zonisamide* finished first, then the *Lacosamide* sometime in the middle of the following year, and finally have the *Oxcarbazepine* tapered off last. So, all three AEDs should be done in a year and a half. That will leave you only on the *Brivaracetam*."

"Okay. I tried to memorize all of what he had said.

"Then, we can start to decrease the *Brivaracetam* next if your body is okay without the other three AEDs. I believe that's the plan we will go with. I don't believe in pulling patients off of medication right away, tapering the medication off is safer which is why it will take longer. But it will be extremely beneficial for you James."

"Okay, that sounds great." I was more than excited for the plan we both made.

"In fact James, since you haven't had any seizures for two months now, I am going to start by lowering your *Zonisamide* today."

I had been shocked to hear that. But I was excited.

"Starting this evening, instead of taking 5 100mg capsules, I want you to take 4 100mg capsules and continue that from now on. So, your new medication list consists of: *Oxcarbazepine* 2 600mg tab/2x daily, *Lacosamide* 1 100mg tab/2x daily, *Brivaracetam* 1 100mg tab 2x/daily, and finally the new dosage, *Zonisamide* changes from 5 to 4 100mg capsules in the evening."

"Okay. I will make sure to do that. I also have a question. I know it's too early to apply, but I wanted to ask."

"Okay, what's your question?"

"How long before I can apply for a driver's license? I know I had a few Focal Seizures."

"So, yes, it's too early for that. However, as long as you haven't had any seizure that have impaired your consciousness, then you are good. So Focal Seizures are actually okay if they are controlled because you are aware and able to control your movement and body. Unlike your previous type of seizure."

"Oh wow, I didn't know that. I thought it was any seizure. So I just have to wait a year from July then?"

"You can actually start applying in the early spring of 2021, I'd say March or even late February. You only need to be eight months without an impaired seizure."

"That makes me happy to hear. I've been waiting an exceedingly long time for that. Thank you for that information."

"Like I said, and Doctor Boden as well, be confident in yourself and start to live life. It's different than you have the past ten years, but your brain will adjust. Again, you have a very bright future ahead of you."

I wanted to cry when he spoke those words, but I held back the emotions I felt.

"I will definitely be confident. Thank you Doctor Devrat."

"Alright James, bye now."

"Bye." We hung up the call that day and I was the happiest I had been in a long time. My hope was a burning passion. I had so much joy, faith, and good news in a matter of days.

VIRTUAL EPILEPSY WALKS – NOVEMBER 2020

I had felt confident in not only myself, but also my health and life. By the time November had

arrived, it was time for the two Epilepsy walks I had signed up for. The first walk took place on

November 7. My healing had been going well, and I exercised five to six days a week, so I

walked three miles for that walk. On November 15, the second walk, I had already added

weightlifting to my exercise routine, as it hadn't overexerted my brain, so I walked four miles.

For both walks, I had been sent a printable sign. The sign read, *I walk for*, and on it I

wrote: *Myself and Everyone who Battles Epilepsy.* My purpose I had for the two walks was to

advocate and be a shining beacon of hope for those with the chronic illness that once filled my

life, and almost took it at one point. To let them know there was more than just despair and

JAMES VALENCIA

Darkness, which I myself had seen for so long.

When I had finished both walks on the days, I went to my bedroom where I logged into my laptop to video call with the other groups and people who had also walked. I had also talked with the sponsors who supported the walks. It was a great way of connecting with the different people, as we all had different stories of how it led us to Epilepsy.

I knew after those walks and having talked to the members and sponsors that I wanted to advocate for as long as I could for people like myself and who still struggled. I knew what it was like to struggle, and I wasn't going to stop advocating and fighting until we found a cure and ways to help.

. . . . .

But I trust in your unfailing Love;

my heart rejoices in your salvation.

I will sing the Lord's praise,

for He has been good to me.

PSALMS 13:5-6

322

EPILOGUE

Sometimes I lay in bed at night thinking about the original diagnosis of my illness. I just stare at my ceiling only to recall the memories of past trauma that had occurred throughout my journey with Epilepsy. I recall it so vividly it taunts me. It's almost like Satan himself is reminding me of the loneliness and sadness I once I had. The very thing that threatened my life towards the end of my Epilepsy diagnosis was still there in the room, reminding me of the shame I once had.

But then I hear a voice. A gentle, loving voice whispers into my ears, "You are not there anymore my child. Do not let this demon and monster fool you. I have brought you up from the ashes you once were." I smile, only to know and be reminded that through the tough and difficult journey I endured, God had been there. He had placed me on the difficult path so I could meet the friends, professors, and colleagues I have today. All I needed to do was trust in Him, although it would take me over nine and a half years to do so. He had a purpose for my journey, through the darkness I had felt for so long.

I think about how I tried to hide my Epilepsy from my professors at the college. How I would lock myself away in the practice rooms and never make friends for months my freshman year but was unsuccessful. Then finally, Dr. Anders and Dr. Marino sat down with me to reassure me that I was safe to not be judged by them or the students at the school. That it was okay to have a health problem, to be different and myself.

The night the music fraternity showed me so much compassion and love I could never forget. When I had the seizure at the softball field my sophomore year of college, and was ashamed to tell anyone, but the fraternity welcomed me with open arms. "Jimmy, you are not a burden. We love you Brother."

The thought of all the AED medication I had tried. I always wondered why it never worked. *Why hadn't it worked for me? Of all people, am I just that unlucky?* But no, there was a purpose. A mission at the end I was going to accomplish. Or I think of Doctor Klark, and how he wasn't able to help me, but it was meant to be. It was to help me get into the *Medical Center*. If it weren't for the *Medical Center*, the cluster seizures I was having could've taken my very own life.

The worst thought I think about at night, as I lay in bed staring at the ceiling, is when I was told about my Intractable Epilepsy. It felt like someone had told me I was dying. "There's nothing else we can do for your Epilepsy. No other medications we can give you. Have you considered surgery? If we don't control your seizures, it can lead to serious injury and possibly... death." It broke my heart hearing those words spoken aloud that December of 2019.

But then, as I lay in my bed, I hear the voice whisper again. "Son, remember what happens next in your story." And I smile. After that appointment in December of 2019, I went home and locked myself in my room where I cried. And for the first time in nine and a half years I fell to my knees and said out loud to God on that rainy day, "God, I give up. I'm scared. There is nothing the doctors have left for me but possibly brain surgery. Please, I need you. Wherever you are if you can hear me. Whatever happens next in this long road ahead of me, I trust you. I fully trust you with all of my heart. I'm broken. I can't do this without you."

I thank God every day for what has occurred in my life over my journey with Epilepsy. No, it hasn't been an easy road and I sometimes wish it hadn't occurred. But I thank Him all the time for choosing me and not my sisters to endure the challenges I faced. I wouldn't have been able to bear watching them suffer the way I did. The lonely nights I sat in the college parking lot alone, as I cried out to God wondering when my suffering would end. Other harmful activities I regret, as I tried to numb the pain. But in the end, I thank Him for walking by my side and how He lined everything up perfectly for me. Also, how He gave me friends that were put into my path that I now rely on and will always have. The teachers and professors who never gave up on me, even when I thought they would. How the shimmer of hope that never left my beating heart.

JAMES VALENCIA

God, I know I say it all the time now, but I don't know how to repay you for all you have brought me through over the past ten years. When I saw ashes, You gave me life. I want to bring light and hope to the world. and people who need it.

The purpose of my journey I do not fully understand, and I may never understand. But what I do know is that I am faithfully called to give the hope that was barely left within my own self, to those who struggle with it themselves. It was a difficult task to write the pages contained within this memoir. The many days, months, tears, and prayers of writing were endless. It took all my strength to put my hardships into words, as I tried so hard to forget them. But, as I kept hearing the whisper from my God in my ear to tell my story, I did what I was faithfully asked, and what I felt in my heart to do. So, here I stand, six months post- surgery and seizure free. No more darkness, but instead a beacon of hope for the world to see.

. . . . . .

We have this hope as an anchor for the soul,

firm and secure. It enters the

inner sanctuary behind the curtain.

HEBREWS 6:19

326

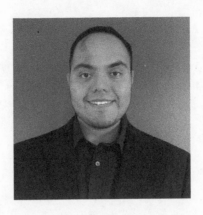

ABOUT THE AUTHOR

JAMES VALENCIA graduated with his Bachelor of Music in Education & Voice Performance, as well as a Master of Arts in Education for Learning & Teaching. He currently sings in a professional choir in Southern California, where he also teaches music and choir.

Valencia devotes his time advocating for Epilepsy awareness and is a strong voice for those in the Epilepsy community. He participates in multiple Walk to End Epilepsy walks to raise awareness, and consistently helps raise funds for different organizations to help find a cure for Epilepsy and seizures.

ABOUT THE BOOK

AT FOURTEEN YEARS OLD and deeply rooted in faith, family, and friends in a small Southern California town, James Valencia was diagnosed with Epilepsy, a seizure and neurological disorder. It seemed like a heavy burden upon his shoulders at such a young age.

As he and his parents tried to get him the medical care he desperately needed, he was put through many Anti-Epileptic medications throughout his journey with Epilepsy. Some failing and other working. The constant torture of never knowing when a seizure would occur overwhelmed him. He needed to choose between giving up his faith and hope or decide whether he was going to trust it would be okay.

By examining the battles of his life over the years he has lived with his diagnosis, James traces the complexity of his health and the journey it has taken him on. He is able to find the love and support within his friends, family, community, and himself. Despite the heartbreaks, tears, and trials he has endured, he finds hope in the shimmer of light barely left for him to see. This memoir is a testament to the love and hope that survives all the battles that were placed upon him.